VALUE-ADDED ROLES for MEDICAL STUDENTS

VALUE-ADDED ROLES for MEDICAL STUDENTS

The AMA MedEd Innovation Series

JED D. GONZALO, MD, MSc

MAYA M. HAMMOUD, MD, MBA

GREGORY W. SCHNEIDER, MD

ELSEVIER

Elsevier
1600 John F. Kennedy Blvd.
Ste 1800
Philadelphia, PA 19103-2899

VALUE-ADDED ROLES FOR MEDICAL STUDENTS

ISBN: 978-0-323-75950-2

Notices

Knowledge and best practice in this field are constantly changing. As new research and experience broaden our understanding, changes in research methods, professional practices, or medical treatment may become necessary.

Practitioners and researchers must always rely on their own experience and knowledge in evaluating and using any information, methods, compounds or experiments described herein. Because of rapid advances in the medical sciences, in particular, independent verification of diagnoses and drug dosages should be made. To the fullest extent of the law, no responsibility is assumed by Elsevier, authors, editors or contributors for any injury and/or damage to persons or property as a matter of products liability, negligence or otherwise, or from any use or operation of any methods, products, instructions, or ideas contained in the material herein.

Library of Congress Control Number: 2021938650

Content Strategist: Elyse O'Grady
Content Development Manager: Ellen Wurm-Cutter
Publishing Services Manager: Deepthi Unni
Project Manager: Janish Ashwin Paul
Design Direction: Patrick Ferguson

Printed in United States

Last digit is the print number: 9   8   7   6   5   4   3   2   1

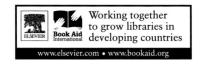

CONTENTS

FOREWORD

The American Medical Association's Accelerating Change in Medical Education Consortium is working to create new approaches to health professions training to ultimately improve patient outcomes. Our consortium has produced significant innovations in a number of areas that are being adopted at multiple schools. To assist in the dissemination of these innovations, we are pleased to present a series of books to aid the adoption of these ideas at additional health professions schools and training programs.

The AMA MedEd Innovation Series provides practical guidance for local implementation of the education innovations tested and refined by the AMA consortium. This AMA *Value-Added Roles for Medical Students: Theory, Practice, and Implementation Guide* is the second in this series. Future subjects will include strategies for creating an academic coaching program, improving change management for faculty, implementing health systems science education, and incorporating the electronic health record into curricula.

The *Value-Added Roles for Medical Students: Theory, Practice, and Implementation Guide* presents the theoretical foundations for value-added roles in undergraduate medical education, approaches for creating program evaluation and assessment tools, seven exemplar programs from around the country, and an overview of the implementation process for a value-added medical education program, including the resources needed and tips for success.

We are pleased to offer this second book in the AMA MedEd Innovation Series and look forward to learning about your experience in implementing value-added roles at your institution.

Susan E. Skochelak, MD, MPH
Chief Academic Officer
American Medical Association

We are pleased to present *Value-Added Roles for Medical Students: Theory, Practice, and Implementation Guide.*

A variety of forces over the last several decades have transformed health systems throughout the United States and beyond. These changes have compelled medical educators to adapt and to reshape the structure and opportunities provided for medical students. Health systems science has emerged as a third pillar of medical education for students and residents as evolving health systems begin to demand that physicians and other health care professionals have "systems-ready" knowledge, attitudes, and skills. Since clinical practice environments are crucial for learning and for professional development, educators have aspired to find roles for students within those environments that provide opportunities both for meaningful contributions to patient care and for learning health systems science. These opportunities represent "value-added roles," in which value is added to the local health care environment and to the students' education.

In 2016, 32 US medical schools in the American Medical Association's Accelerating Change in Medical Education Consortium met for a 2-day national meeting to explore value-added medical education. The participants identified potential stakeholders regarding the value of student work and roles and tasks that students could perform to add value to the health system, including key barriers and associated strategies to promote value-added roles in undergraduate medical education. This book on value-added roles, also the work of the consortium, follows in the tradition of that original meeting.

In Part I, we present the theoretical foundations for value-added roles in undergraduate medical education and approaches for creating program evaluation and assessment tools. Part II showcases seven exemplar programs from around the country, where institutions have successfully launched value-added roles for their students as patient navigators, practice improvement champions, members of microsystems and interprofessional care teams, and more. Part III provides an overview of the implementation process for a value-added medical education program, including the resources needed and tips for success.

We hope you find this book helpful as you seek to explore and launch value-added medical education programs of your own.

Jed D. Gonzalo, MD, MSc
Maya M. Hammoud, MD, MBA
Gregory W. Schneider, MD

ACKNOWLEDGMENTS

The editors and authors of this book would like to thank Sarah Ayala of the American Medical Association (AMA) for her project management. Without her, this book would not exist. We'd like to thank Victoria Stagg Elliott, also of the AMA, for her copyediting and catching our misspellings and misused words. Kevin Heckman of the AMA and director of the AMA MedEd Innovation Series gets our gratitude for his support of this book. We give additional thanks to the members of the AMA Accelerating Change in Medical Education Consortium, who contributed to this book's creation and to Susan E. Skochelak, MD, MPH, the AMA's group vice president for medical education. Without her leadership, the consortium and, thus, this book would not have been possible.

VALUE-ADDED ROLES for MEDICAL STUDENTS

PART I

Theory

Part I, *Theory*, lays out the historical background and conceptual foundations underpinning this book. Topics discussed include the concepts of value-added roles and community of practice; the educational theories involved in value-added medical education; and examples of historical and emerging value-added roles for students. The opening chapter sets the stage by providing an overview of learning opportunities available with value-added roles, with an emphasis on health systems science and the urgent need to expand the educational experience for medical students. This section makes the case for how value-added roles have the potential both to enhance student education and to add value to local health systems. The second chapter offers a historical perspective, describing the evolution of value-added roles for students. The third chapter focuses on competencies, assessment, and program evaluation, with an emphasis on setting up an evaluation plan and using an evaluation framework in order to create a robust ongoing quality improvement process.

1

Concept of Value-Added Roles: Creating a Community of Practice

Jed D. Gonzalo, Gregory W. Schneider, and Daniel R. Wolpaw

LEARNING OBJECTIVES

1. Define value-added roles and tasks for medical students.
2. Describe the evolution of value-added roles and tasks in US medical education and the urgent need to create and expand these critical learning opportunities.
3. Identify key learning areas for students embedded in value-added roles, specifically related to health systems science, clinical science, and health humanities.
4. Situate value-added roles and tasks within the context of educational theories that influence student motivation and engagement in learning, such as communities of practice and Bandura's concept of self-efficacy.

OUTLINE

CHAPTER SUMMARY

In this first chapter, we describe and explore the concept of value-added medical education, which includes the roles and tasks for medical students in clinical workplace environments that can add value to care delivery processes while also allowing students to learn clinical and systems-based competencies. We present several key events within health care delivery that have influenced the role students have in their clinical experiences (e.g., clerkships) and the trend of decreasing responsibility and authentic engagement in the team's work. Using a communities-of-practice conceptual framework, we describe the relationship between students' roles and tasks, their relationship to the health care system and the clinicians within the clinical environment, and the students' engagement and motivation to contribute to patient care and learn new skills. The chapter closes with a brief summary of the subsequent chapters and the proposed ways in which this book can be used by students and educators to advance US medical education.

INTRODUCTION

Medical education is evolving in the context of health care delivery systems facing the complex adaptive challenge of navigating a shifting economic and regulatory landscape while striving to achieve the Triple Aim of the Institute for Healthcare Improvement (IHI): simultaneously improving the patient experience of care and the health of populations while reducing the per capita cost of health care.[1,2] Additionally, some institutions, including the American Medical Association, support expanding the Triple Aim to the Quadruple Aim, which includes improving the work life of physicians and other health care professionals. To remain effective and relevant, medical schools and associated academic health systems must take on the difficult challenge of re-creating curricula to align with the demands of leading and practicing in this transforming care environment.[3] Educating in biomedical science is necessary but no longer sufficient. Graduating students need to understand and function in a changed and changing health care world. We believe success in this process will depend on whether education leaders can successfully address two unmet needs: (1) creating learning experiences that add value to health systems and (2) prioritizing and improving education for future physicians in health systems science (HSS), which includes concepts such as population and public health, health systems improvement, and value-based care.[3,4] This textbook, written by leaders at US medical schools, provides a re-envisioning of "value-added medical education" as an opportunity to create experiences for students that both add value to the health system and enhance education in HSS. We anticipate that this book will move the conversation forward and provide guidance as we all work to educate the physician workforce in a way that will advance the care of patients and populations in this century.

THE URGENT NEED

Over the last 50 years, the ways in which medical students have been able to contribute to health care delivery have changed. In the early years of the 20th century, medical students in academic health centers were often relegated to very peripheral roles. This status shifted over time, particularly in the face of wartime workforce shortages, when students helped fill various gaps in care.[5] Student contributions to patient care were relied on to help meet unfilled needs—the roles and tasks performed by the students were "value added" to the care delivery processes. They assisted residents in performing many routine tasks and responsibilities on hospital-based wards, including dressing changes, blood draws, electrocardiograms, and charting. They were often viewed as part of the team. Physicians and other health care professionals depended on students to lighten the load and support essential care. These were authentic roles that were routinely "paid forward" by educational efforts from appreciative residents and staff, and they truly added value for patients, caregivers, and students.

Over the past several decades, student opportunities to contribute to the daily work of patient care have significantly declined. Legal, financial, and regulatory oversight instituted to improve and standardize care has reframed many former student activities as "high stakes" and severely curtailed student ability to make meaningful contributions to health care teams.[6,7] Today, students in both the preclerkship and clerkship environments enter clinical rotations mainly as observers. They are linked with attending physicians to watch, learn, and eventually practice "doctoring skills" (e.g., history and physical examination), professionalism, and key aspects of the doctor-patient relationship. This apprenticeship approach to clinical experiences requires time and skill on the part of faculty physicians to appropriately mentor and educate students. This process can decrease the faculty physician's clinical efficiency and negatively impact productivity, thereby creating tension about the student's presence in the clinical environment.[8] As a result, nearly all student work is relegated to a peripheral and nonessential role on the health care team. In this paradigm, learners can become valued contributors to teams only when they finally are able to make independent, clinically based decisions, such as making a diagnosis or therapeutic plan—and this level of autonomy comes only after considerable practice and training. This transition to "physician contributor" takes years to achieve and usually does not occur until residency.

ARE MEDICAL STUDENTS AN ASSET OR A LIABILITY?

With the advent of increasing productivity pressures, oversight regulations, liability concerns, and the associated decline in opportunities for students to make meaningful contributions, the impact of medical student education on the function of care teams has come under increasing scrutiny (Fig. 1.1). The dominant apprenticeship model requires clinical settings, and health care leaders are faced with questions of how to limit cost and improve efficiency within those same clinical learning environments. Several studies, although dated, suggest that the time dedicated by faculty physicians in the teaching of medical students, as well as graduate trainees, significantly limits their clinical efficiency and productivity. By some estimates, the overall cost may increase by 25%, well in excess of the student tuition.[9] In addition, several studies estimate that student presence in an outpatient clinic can add up to 60 minutes of additional work for the faculty preceptor each day.[10]

Based on the historical narrative and these practice-based studies, it is fair to suggest that over the last half century the asset-to-liability balance for medical students has shifted.

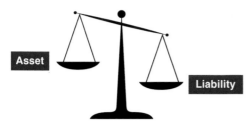

Fig. 1.1 Are Medical Students in Today's Clinical Environments an Asset or Liability to Care? This question is critical for today's US medical schools and academic health centers, particularly in a time of increasing productivity pressures for physicians and decreasing autonomy of student work.

This observation is not simply academic—it is a critical challenge in medical education. Learners who are viewed and view themselves as active contributors to their community of practice have the opportunity to experience the kind of engagement and motivation that is essential to professional development. This is a complex adaptive challenge that will not be solved by tinkering with old models. We believe the answer lies in the evolution of our understanding of the determinants of health and disease, in the increasing efforts of health systems to address that understanding, and in the capability of our students to contribute in this transforming landscape. A new approach to creating authentic, meaningful student roles requires shifts in the mindsets of multiple stakeholders in medical education and care delivery systems. In this book, we propose to conceptualize and advance the idea of value-added medical education, education that creates roles and tasks that add value to the health care system and where students are truly seen as assets.

WHAT ARE THE WAYS MEDICAL STUDENTS CAN ADD VALUE?

When student roles are considered primarily from the perspective of a passive apprenticeship model, it is much harder to imagine how they might add value to the care environment. Consequently, it is critical to frame the creation of value-added educational opportunities as a complex adaptive challenge, accessing multiple perspectives. These diverse points of view not only open up fresh ideas but also support meaningful alignment between education, health care delivery systems, and the needs of patients and populations (Table 1.1).[11,12] We anticipate that this matrix of perspectives will be helpful to curriculum developers and health system leaders as they design, implement, and evaluate new or evolved value-added roles and programs.

Perspectives to Consider

Patients—The patients within our health systems can potentially benefit from the contributions of students, improving their care experiences and outcomes.

Clinical educators and teachers—Although, as noted, some studies suggest that student presence tends to "slow down" preceptors in clinical settings, there are also some emerging strategies for how students can be positioned to improve preceptor efficiency. In addition, many preceptors find joy and satisfaction in educating the next generation of physicians.

Clinical site—Embedded students can be assigned to work on improving care processes, outcomes (e.g., population health initiatives), or community-based outreach.

Hospital or academic health center—Several possible benefits can be imagined. (1) Meaningful student integration into care delivery processes can benefit health care systems through a range of often underresourced roles (aspects of discharge communication, coordination with community organizations and resources, etc.). (2) Student engagement and service-learning projects can support partnerships with outreach programs or other local organizations. A hospital, for instance, might partner with a local community farm and offer a food prescription program, with students playing an integral role in the program's operation. (3) Many patients prefer to receive care at an academic hospital where teaching is a primary focus.

Medical students—Students integrated into value-added roles and tasks within clinical practice sites can benefit by experiencing and solidifying new clinical and HSS competencies as well as by developing their professional identities as authentic participants in health care teams.

Medical educators—The faculty physicians working with students in roles/tasks that are designed to meaningfully contribute to patient care can benefit from improving their coaching skills and gaining new knowledge and skill expertise, particularly in the areas of HSS. A more knowledgeable cohort of frontline educators can accelerate the change needed in medical education to best prepare learners to improve patient outcomes.

Medical school—Creating meaningful value-added roles for students aligns with the best education science, supports a culture of innovation and educational leadership, strengthens mutually beneficial relationships with the health system, and advances the vision of graduating physicians who will be prepared to thrive in complex, changing environments and improve the health of patients and populations.

TABLE 1.1	Stakeholders, Benefits, and Costs of Value-Added Roles in Health Systems		
Stakeholders		**Benefit**	**Cost**
Health system	Patient(s)	• Improved outcomes • Improved patient experience • Lower utilization of resources or costs of care	• Discomfort or dissatisfaction with student program • Stress or discomfort with process
	Clinical educators	• Improved work efficiency • Gratification in fulfilling social responsibility of student education • Improved work experience	• Reduced clinical productivity • Additional resources needed • Concerns regarding quality of mentoring roles
	Clinical or community site	• Enhanced quality improvement programs and resources • Enhanced partnerships with community resource programs	• Resources and time required for student presence and work
	Hospital system	• Improved relationships with community and neighboring health systems • Improved efficiency through optimal use of students and sparing other human resources	• Time and resources to fund programs
Educational system	Learners	• Improved knowledge, skills, and attitudes in HSS • Improved attitudes of professional role identity • Improved attitudes related to change agency potential • Improved intrinsic motivation for career development • Greater sense of civic responsibility for medical profession	• Competing demands of other courses • Competing demands of licensing examinations • Apprehension and anxiety from performing patient-centered tasks
	Medical educators	• Improved knowledge and skills in HSS, thereby increasing education for other learners	• Investment in learning new concepts
	Medical school	• Enhanced knowledge and skills in new initiative • Creation of educationally meaningful clinical work for medical students • Enhanced credibility in fulfilling social commitment to the community	• Competing demands of other curricular initiatives • Additional faculty and staff time to direct program

HSS, Health systems science.

From Gonzalo JD, Dekhtyar M, Hawkins RE, Wolpaw DR. How can medical students add value? Identifying Roles, Barriers, and Strategies to Advance the Value of Undergraduate medical education to patient care and the health system. *Acad Med.* 2017;92(9):1294–1301. doi:10.1097/acm.0000000000001662
A portion of this framework was informed by the work of Ogrinc et al.[12]

Define Value-Added Roles and Tasks for Medical Students

Within the context of these different perspectives on how medical students can add value, the primary focus of this textbook is on patient care and student education. Students arrive in medical school with remarkable capabilities and a drive to begin to engage in their profession. Traditional curriculum approaches largely ignore these attributes, focusing on content learning and clinical skills for up to 2 years. Students enter their clerkships anxious to apply their nascent physician skills but often missing the same engagement and excitement they brought to medical school.[13] The reality is that entrustment in patient care activities need not wait until the latter years of medical school—and can occur within the first month. In recent years, medical educators and system leaders have been recommending and articulating the ways in which students can actively contribute to care delivery, particularly through experiential learning opportunities.[6] The concept of "value-added medical education" balances student education with the potential to contribute to systems of care. Value-added medical education is defined as:

> Medical student roles that are experiential and authentic and have the potential to have a positive impact on individual and population health outcomes, costs of care, or other processes within the health care system, while also enhancing student knowledge, attitudes, and skills in the clinical or health systems sciences.[8]

CONCEPTUAL FRAMEWORKS FOR VALUE-ADDED ROLES AND TASKS

Several conceptual frameworks are helpful to support and expand our understanding of value-added roles and tasks in the context of medical education. Fig. 1.2 depicts the relationship of traditional US medical student roles and the interprofessional team members working together to improve the health of patients. The patient is at the center of a process that features clinician skill and expertise integrated into a collaborative care team.[8]

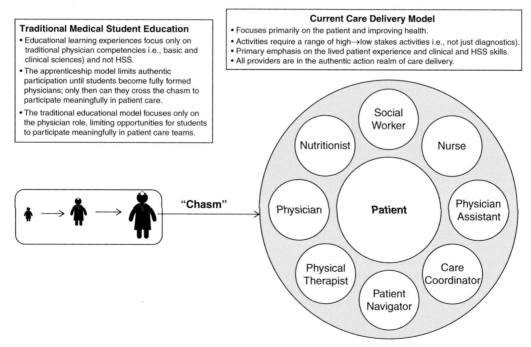

Fig. 1.2 Conceptual Schematic of the Current Chasm Between Traditional Physician-Centric Medical Education and the Current Care Delivery Models. (From Gonzalo JD, Thompson BM, Haidet P, Mann K, Wolpaw DR. A constructive reframing of student roles and systems learning in medical education using a communities of practice lens. *Acad Med.* 2017;92(12):1687–1694. doi:10.1097/acm.0000000000001778.)

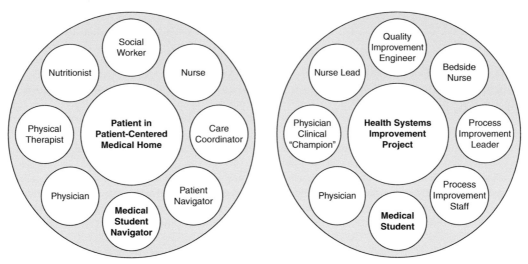

Fig. 1.3 Examples of Value-Added Roles for Medical Students. In the first example, students can be embedded onto primary-care teams in outpatient settings. Specific tasks include speaking with patients, identifying underlying barriers to care, targeting specific interventions to overcome barriers, facilitating communication with clinic staff, and identifying areas for improvement within the clinic. Student supervision and mentorship can be administered by a myriad of providers rather than the requirement for the physician as a lead mentor. In the second example, students can be embedded into quality improvement teams to contribute to ongoing performance improvement. Specific tasks can include interviewing frontline staff about root causes of an issue, challenges/barriers preventing improvement, brainstorming improvement strategies, and contributing to improvement plans. Supervision and mentorship can be administered by a myriad of providers, including quality improvement staff. (From Gonzalo JD, Thompson BM, Haidet P, Mann K, Wolpaw DR. A constructive reframing of student roles and systems learning in medical education using a communities of practice lens. *Acad Med.* 2017;92(12):1687–1694. doi:10.1097/acm.0000000000001778.)

In the apprenticeship model (left side of Fig. 1.2), medical students are educated in a "mini-physician" pathway. Students shadow attending physicians, view the health system from a physician-centric lens, and enter the clinical community of practice care team only after competence is attained, that is, after years of education. However, we are entering an era of more complex care coordination, driven not only by quality and safety considerations but also by the multifaceted needs of patients and populations. There is an increasing focus on interprofessional collaborative care teams and awareness of the need to proactively address social, financial, and logistical barriers in patients' health care. In this context, we believe that medical students can enter the wheel hub and become contributing team members early in medical school by simultaneously learning and performing meaningful health care tasks (Fig. 1.3). Students can experience authentic collaboration rather than merely observing or studying the process in a classroom, relating to the physician within the team as a colleague rather than as an apprentice. In addition, because the interdependent team members are actual contributors to the health system, students have the opportunity to make legitimate contributions and improve patient health. We imagine a world where the absence of a medical student on a team is seen as an adverse event that leads to poorer team functioning rather than the current model in which student presence is often viewed as a burden to team functioning (through increased load on the system).

There are several opportunities for students to assume value-added roles as patient navigators, health coaches, quality improvement team members, or emergency medical technicians (two examples are shown in Fig. 1.3). These roles add value to clinical sites and programs as "force multipliers" for nonphysician roles, such as care managers and coordinators. Students can also provide services not typically offered in certain settings through patient education, psychological or emotional support, or assistance in facilitating access to care or resources. In these roles, students can contribute to the team in a way that aligns with current health system needs, including reducing readmissions, improving care transitions, and improving patient health and satisfaction. We propose that by moving toward these kinds of value-added roles, students can authentically contribute their knowledge, attitudes, and skills to the health care system while learning HSS-related concepts.

EDUCATIONAL BENEFITS—HEALTH SYSTEMS SCIENCE AS A "PASSPORT" INTO VALUE-ADDED ROLES

As team-based care models evolve in US health care delivery, we believe now is the time for exploring ways in which medical student roles can add value to health systems while developing the knowledge, skills, and mindset of future physicians in systems-based learning.[14] Over the past 30 years, policy makers, educators, system leaders, and students have been calling for additional focus on learning about care systems and

better aligning medical education with the needs of patients and health systems. In response to these recommendations, the "third science" of HSS (in addition to basic and clinical sciences), has been established as a comprehensive framework to accelerate change.[3,14] HSS provides a necessary foundation for the successful application of biomedical science and for realizing the vision of IHI's Triple Aim. HSS includes concepts such as population health, health care policy, systems thinking, economics, cost-conscious and high-value care, health system improvement, and interprofessional teamwork. It provides new opportunities for medical students to develop important knowledge, attitudes, and skills that do not necessarily require high-stakes medical diagnostics and therapeutics.

The HSS framework (Fig. 1.4) cohesively unites a previously scattered collection of systems-related

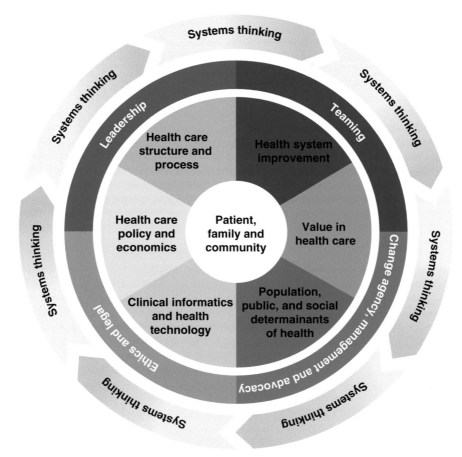

Fig. 1.4 The Health Systems Science Framework. This figure depicts the 12 distinct competency domains for health systems science (HSS). The six internal pie pieces include the core competency areas, while the four domains around the circle include the cross-cutting domains. Systems thinking encircles all the pieces, demonstrating the cohesive and all-encompassing role this competency domain serves in the HSS framework. Patient, family, and community, of course, are at the center. (Reprinted with permission of the American Medical Association. ©Copyright American Medical Association 2020. All rights reserved.)

competencies.[15] It is now being used by several dozen undergraduate medical education (UME) and graduate medical education (GME) programs, and currently informs several national initiatives. Many of the HSS competencies have been a part of medical education for years, such as the Accreditation Council for Graduate Medical Education (ACGME) Systems-Based Practice (SBP) Competency. However, medical education continues to experience significant challenges in implementing and operationalizing these systems-based learning areas.[16,17] The HSS-related competencies are often relegated to peripheral pockets of the curriculum and depend heavily on local contexts, including curricular priorities and available expertise. This "add-on" approach contributes to fragmented learning for medical students, which we believe compromises their professional development and limits their impact on patient health. Studies also suggest that US medical students are noticing these gaps, reporting inadequate education in health care systems, economics, managed care, and practice management.

Value-added roles and tasks are a primary means through which to operationalize HSS learning and professional development. Within weeks of starting medical school, students can partner with nonphysician health care professionals to make authentic and meaningful contributions at a time when they are just beginning on the path to traditional doctoring competencies. As part of national efforts to promote education in HSS, many US medical schools are developing these experiential opportunities with the goals of (1) advancing learning in HSS; (2) building foundations in clinical science; and (3) perhaps most importantly, supporting a process of professional identity formation that reflects our transforming health care world (see subsequent chapters in this textbook). We also believe that these early opportunities to connect with functioning health care teams and make a difference for patients in need validate and stimulate student motivation for learning HSS.

Several studies have demonstrated this alignment of value-added roles with learning in HSS. At Penn State College of Medicine (see Chapter 4) for example, medical students are embedded into interprofessional care sites as patient navigators. These students report extensive learning in both HSS and clinical skills, including interprofessional collaboration, communication, the context of health care delivery systems, high-value care, and social determinants of health. We believe that these kinds of authentic, contributory experiences are key to the professional development of "collaboratively effective, systems-ready physicians."[18]

Clinical Vignette

A year one medical student working as a patient navigator is assigned to the physical medicine and rehabilitation hospital. In her role, she is assigned to be mentored by a faculty member who is the care coordinator. The student patient navigator role is to extend the clinical team and perform a number of activities that help the patient reach the desired outcomes while the student is still learning. Some of the student's tasks include performing home safety assessments for patients who are scheduled to be discharged. Many of these patients have new functional requirements, and their homes may need new features to ensure safety, continued recovery, and sufficient functional ability. Additionally, the patient may have several social determinants of health that need to be addressed by the care team for an optimal discharge and transition. The student patient navigator is assigned new patients and reviews all of the relevant data pertaining to the patient's case in the electronic health record. This is followed by an interview with the patient to build a trusting relationship, identify any needs the patient may have, and begin the home assessment. After meeting with the patient in the rehab hospital prior to discharge, the student performs a home visit with a classmate (or another clinical team member). Following the interview and visit, the student patient navigator documents the encounters in the electronic health record, identifying any potential gaps in care or patient needs and the plans for addressing those needs. The student then presents the patient's case during an interprofessional care team huddle.

This scenario illustrates how a medical student can become part of an interprofessional care team within a clinical site to assist patients with their needs and extend the work of the care team while learning. Through these experiences, the learning includes a breadth of competencies, ranging from taking a history, including social determinants of health, to documenting in the electronic health record as well as beginning to develop competencies in transitions of care, patient safety, interprofessional collaboration, professionalism, and systems thinking (Table 1.2).

A NEW PROFESSIONAL IDENTITY AS SYSTEMS CITIZENS

The complexity of the current health care environment and advances in our understanding of the science of health and disease are requiring a re-examination of what it means to

TABLE 1.2   The Competency Grid for Value-Added Roles

Health Systems Science Areas	Competency in Value-Added Role
Patient experience and context • Patient experience and values • Patient behaviors and motivations	X
Health care delivery • Structures of delivery • Processes of delivery	X
Health care policy and economics • Policy • Economics and payment	X
Population, public, and social determinants of health • Social determinants of health • Public health • Population health and improvement	X
Clinical informatics and health technology • Informatics/data analytics • Decision support/evidence-based medicine • Technology and tools	X
Value in health care • Quality principles and dimensions • Cost and waste • Evaluation/metrics	X
Health system improvement • Improvement principles, processes, and tools • Data and measurement • Innovation and scholarship	
Systems thinking	X
Change agency, management, and advocacy	X
Ethics and legal	
Leadership	
Teaming and teamwork	X
Clinical Science	
Effectively manage communication with patients/interprofessional care team.	X
Comprehensively assess and diagnose the root causes of patients' situations.	X
Build a therapeutic relationship with a patient.	X
Professionalism	
Interact professionally with patients, staff, and clinicians in informal and clinically based settings.	X
Document patient encounters in the electronic health record in a timely and accurate manner.	X
Participate in and contribute to the ongoing work of an interprofessional care team.	X
Demonstrate practice-based learning strategies for continuous long-term growth.	X

be a physician and healer. There is an evolving consensus that traditional biomedical expertise alone is necessary but not sufficient to address the health needs of patients and populations. In 2013, Catherine Lucey advocated that medical education pivot from training "personally expert sovereign physicians" to developing "collaboratively effective systems physicians."[19] There is a growing consensus that although the need for physician expertise continues, the aperture through which we view professional identity needs to grow and adapt to the health care environment (or "country") where we live and work. We need to think about what it means to be an engaged citizen of that country—a systems citizen.[20-22] Originally articulated by Peter Senge, systems citizens build genuine partnerships across boundaries, see patterns of interdependency, discern how a system is functioning, and connect with others to engage in a process aimed at achieving outcomes.[23] They not only care for individual patients but also know how to perform in developing systems of care and embody the motivation to grow and contribute to the emergence and evolution of the health care system itself. Just as "digital natives" are individuals born and raised in the culture and language of information technology, we envision medical students engaging in authentic, formative collaboration that will make them "HSS natives" fluent in the language and culture of the health care system and interprofessional collaboration.[24]

CONCLUSION AND FOLLOWING CHAPTERS

The opportunity for medical students to add value to health systems and patients while learning and growing as collaborative health care professionals lies at the intersection of transforming systems of care, advances in medical education, and the evolution of physician professional identity. Leveraging the enormous potential of this opportunity requires a new vision informed by systems thinking and the emerging field of health systems science. Subsequent chapters have been designed to provide tangible strategies, examples, and guideposts for moving this important agenda forward.

TAKE-HOME POINTS

1. There is an urgent need to ensure that medical students engage in meaningful clinical work that contributes to patient care and augments their own education. Many student experiences are too often at the periphery, in nonessential clinical roles.
2. From day one of medical school, students can engage in patient-based experiences that help them to learn about health systems science, the complexity of health care

delivery, and the needs of patients while making a difference and adding value to patient care and contributing to health systems.
3. Communities of practice and self-efficacy can serve as helpful conceptual frameworks for envisioning and designing value-added student roles.
4. Widespread acceptance of the Institute for Healthcare Improvement's Triple Aim and population health improvement should serve as cornerstones of mission and planning for academic health centers. Incorporation of these cornerstones creates the opportunity for experiential educational activities that are cocreated and aligned with systems of care.
5. The concept of systems citizenship encapsulates the needs and aspirations of evolving professionalism and professional identity in a transforming care environment.

QUESTIONS FOR FURTHER THOUGHT

1. How can we accelerate a culture change from the traditional pathway of siloed physician professional development to a collaborative, experiential pathway that incorporates the concept of systems citizenship?
2. How can we create clinical learning environments that support and validate this evolving vision of professional identity?
3. How can we best encourage medical educators and local health systems to incorporate students in meaningful ways in clinical care enterprises?
4. How can we reduce barriers and improve incentives for educators and clinicians to include health systems science more systematically throughout the medical school curriculum?
5. Are there ways to advocate for a more unified effort across the nation in terms of curriculum or assessment to foster the creation of value-added educational experiences for students rather than each school inventing its own process?

ANNOTATED BIBLIOGRAPHY

Dornan T, Boshuizen H, King N, Scherpbier A. Experience-based learning: a model linking the processes and outcomes of medical students' workplace learning. *Med Educ.* 2007;41(1):84–91. https://doi.org/10.1111/j.1365-2929.2006.02652.x.
This seminal article highlights the ways in which opportunities for authentic experiential learning in medical education have changed over time. The authors provide a model for effective workplace learning and advocate for what they call "supported participation," in which students gain practical competence while being given the assistance and resources needed to acquire confidence, motivation, and a sense of professional identity.

Gonzalo JD, Thompson BM, Haidet P, Mann K, Wolpaw DR. A constructive reframing of student roles and systems learning in medical education using a communities of practice lens. *Acad Med.* 2017;92(12):1687–1694. https://doi.org/10.1097/ACM.0000000000001778.

Using key features of community-of-practice theory, the authors contrast current and new experiential learning roles for medical students. They propose the concept of "value-added clinical systems learning roles" as a way to provide students with opportunities to make meaningful contributions to patient care while learning health systems science at the patient and population level.

Gonzalo JD, Dekhtyar M, Hawkins RE, Wolpaw DR. How can medical students add value? Identifying roles, barriers, and strategies to advance the value of undergraduate medical education to patient care and the health system. *Acad Med.* 2017;92(9):1294–1301. https://doi.org/10.1097/ACM.0000000000001662.

This article summarizes takeaways from a 2016 American Medical Association Accelerating Change in Medical Education conference, in which participants met to explore value-added medical education. The conference of educators, AMA staff, students, and systems leaders identified potential new learning roles for students and noted six priority areas for advancing value-added medical education.

Gonzalo JD, Graaf D, Johannes B, Blatt B, Wolpaw DR. Adding value to the health care system: identifying value-added systems roles for medical students. *Am J Med Qual.* 2017;32(3):261–270. https://doi.org/10.1177/1062860616645401.

This study provides the results of a two-year investigation. The investigators toured multiple clinical sites and interviewed stakeholders for their perceptions and ideas with regard to enhanced systems roles for students at their sites. Thematic analysis revealed potential new categories of new systems roles, anticipated benefits for clinics and students, and the elements of a framework for value-added student roles.

Gonzalo JD, Graaf D, Ahluwalia A, Wolpaw DR, Thompson BM. A practical guide for implementing and maintaining value-added clinical systems learning roles for medical students using a diffusion of innovations framework. *Adv Health Sci Educ.* 2018;23(4):699–720. https://doi.org/10.1007/s10459-018-9822-5.

Utilizing a diffusions-of-innovations framework, the authors explore and identify barriers, facilitators, and best practices for implementing value-added clinical systems learning roles for medical students. They identified six important factors that influence program implementation and maintenance, including educational benefit, value added to patient care, student engagement, and mentor time and site capacity.

REFERENCES

1. Porter ME. What Is Value in Health Care? *N Engl J Med.* 2010;363(26):2477–2481.
2. Berwick DM, Nolan TW, Whittington J. The triple aim: care, health, and cost. *Health Aff (Millwood).* 2008;27(3):759–769.
3. Gonzalo JD, Haidet P, Papp KK, et al. Educating for the 21st-century health care system: an interdependent framework of basic, clinical, and systems sciences. *Acad Med.* 2017;92(1):35–39.
4. Skochelak S, Hammoud M, Lomis K, et al. *Health Systems Science.* 2nd ed. Philadelphia, PA: Elsevier; 2020.
5. Ludmerer KM. *Time to Heal: American Medical Education from the Turn of the Century to the Era of Managed Care.* Oxford, NY: Oxford University Press; 1999.
6. Curry RH. Meaningful roles for medical students in the provision of longitudinal patient care. *JAMA.* 2014;312(22):2335–2336.
7. Lin SY, Schillinger E, Irby DM. Value-added medical education: engaging future doctors to transform health care delivery today. *J Gen Intern Med.* 2015;30(2):150–151.
8. Gonzalo JD, Thompson BM, Haidet P, Mann K, Wolpaw DR. A constructive reframing of student roles and systems learning in medical education using a communities of practice lens. *Acad Med.* 2017;92(12):1687–1694. https://doi.org/10.1097/acm.0000000000001778.
9. Jones RF, Korn D. On the cost of educating a medical student. *Acad Med.* 1997;72(3):200–210.
10. Shea S, Nickerson KG, Tenenbaum J, et al. Compensation to a department of medicine and its faculty members for the teaching of medical students and house staff. *N Engl J Med.* 1996;334(3):162–167.
11. Gonzalo JD, Dekhtyar M, Hawkins RE, Wolpaw DR. How can medical students add value? Identifying roles, barriers, and strategies to advance the value of undergraduate medical education to patient care and the health system. *Acad Med.* 2017;92(9):1294–1301. https://doi.org/10.1097/acm.0000000000001662.
12. Ogrinc GS, Headrick LA, Boex JR. Understanding the value added to clinical care by educational activities. Value of Education Research Group. *Acad Med.* 1999;74(10):1080–1086.
13. Yardley S, Littlewood S, Margolis SA, et al. What has changed in the evidence for early experience? Update of a BEME systematic review. *Med Teach.* 2010;32(9):740–746. https://doi.org/10.3109/0142159x.2010.496007.
14. Gonzalo JD, Dekhtyar M, Starr SR, et al. Health systems science curricula in undergraduate medical education. *Acad Med.* 2017;92(1):123–131. https://doi.org/10.1097/acm.0000000000001177.
15. Gonzalo JD, Chang A, Dekhtyar M, Starr SR, Holmboe E, Wolpaw DR. Health systems science in medical education: Unifying the components to catalyze transformation. *Acad Med.* 2020 Sep;95(9):1362–1372. https://doi.org/10.1097/ACM.0000000000003400.
16. Gonzalo JD, Ogrinc G. Health systems science: the "broccoli" of undergraduate medical education. *Acad Med.* 2019;94(10):1425–1432. https://doi.org/10.1097/acm.0000000000002815.
17. Gonzalo JD, Caverzagie KJ, Hawkins RE, Lawson L, Wolpaw DR, Chang A. Concerns and responses for integrating health systems science into medical education. *Acad Med.* 2018;93(6):843–849.

18. Gonzalo JD, Wolpaw D, Graaf D, Thompson BM. Educating patient-centered, systems-aware physicians: a qualitative analysis of medical student perceptions of value-added clinical systems learning roles. *BMC Med Educ.* 2018;18(1):248.

19. Lucey CR. Medical education: part of the problem and part of the solution. *JAMA Intern Med.* 2013;173(17): 1639–1643.

20. Gonzalo JD. Singh MK. Building systems citizenship in health professions education: the continued call for health systems science curricula. *AHRQ PSNet.* https://psnet. ahrq.gov/perspective/building-systems-citizenship-health-professions-education-continued-call-health-systems. Published February 1, 2019. Accessed December 17, 2020.

21. Davis CR, Gonzalo JD. How medical schools can promote community collaboration through health systems science education. *AMA J Ethics.* 2019;21(3):E239–E247.

22. Gonzalo JD, Wolpaw T, Wolpaw D. Curricular transformation in health systems science. *Acad Med.* 2018;93(10):1431–1433. https://doi.org/10.1097/acm.0000000000002284.

23. Senge PM. Systems citizenship: the leadership mandate for this millennium. *Reflections.* 2006;7(3):1–8. https://www.conservationgateway.org/ConservationPlanning/cbd/guidance-document/key-advances/Documents/Systems%20Citizenship_The%20Leadership%20Mandate%20for%20this%20Millenium.pdf. Accessed December 17, 2020.

24. Prensky M. Digital Natives, Digital Immigrants Part 1. *On the Horizon.* 2001;9(5):1–6.

2

Current and Emerging Models

Gregory W. Schneider, Anna Chang, and Jed D. Gonzalo

LEARNING OBJECTIVES

1. Describe ways in which medical students historically have added value to patient care and health systems.
2. Introduce emerging ways in which medical students can add value as part of integrated approaches to patient care and health systems.
3. Identify priority areas for consideration when designing value-added roles for students.
4. Highlight example US programs that offer robust value-added preclerkship, clerkship, and longitudinal experiences for medical students.

OUTLINE

CHAPTER SUMMARY

In this chapter, we draw attention to the ways medical students historically have added value to patient care and health systems and emerging ways students can play more robust value-added roles. Traditional value-added roles include undertaking health system and community health research projects; gathering detailed histories to identify social determinants of health, patient strengths, and barriers to care; and identifying evidence-based interventions at the point of care. Emerging roles include acting as patient navigators and care coordinators, overseeing clinical quality improvement endeavors, participating in longitudinal service-learning enterprises, and contributing to community health activities in diverse clinical care settings. We close with an emphasis on priority areas of consideration for educators hoping to borrow from or implement these examples at their home institutions.

INTRODUCTION

The previous chapter provided definitions of value-added education and roles for medical students. This chapter builds on those definitions, providing a historical context for such roles. It highlights traditional ways medical students have added value within different health care settings and emerging ways medical educators have transformed those experiences, or provided new ones, for medical students. It introduces a handful of exemplary programs in the US that offer robust opportunities for students to engage in value-added roles. Finally, it offers an overview of crucial areas for consideration for medical educators contemplating, or in the midst of implementing, clinical systems learning roles for their students.

Current health systems face pressures to transform at new levels since the explosion of technology and the initiation of Medicare and Medicaid in the 1960s. Today's systems are grappling with increasing accountability for quality of care and are redesigning practice environments to optimize care processes, better align with payment models, and ultimately improve outcomes for patients.[1] The Triple Aim of enhancing the patient experience, improving population health, and reducing costs has become the driver of many of these health care transformations.[2] Additionally, some organizations have expanded the Triple Aim to the Quadruple Aim, which usually includes physician and health care professional wellness. In response, health systems have launched new models, including interprofessional care teams. Medical schools are partnering with those health systems, seeking to foster long-term success by enhancing student engagement in **value-added roles**.[3–8]

These changes have crucial implications for medical educators, as evolving health systems are beginning to demand that physicians and other health care professionals have "systems-ready" knowledge, skills, and attitudes, and because clinical practice environments play such a key role in professional development.[9] Within these environments, the concepts of value-added medical education, value-added student roles, and **health systems science** (HSS) are emerging as increasingly important.[10,11] There is a pressing need for medical schools and health professions programs to transform education to more effectively align with evolving health systems, preparing health care providers who can practice flexibly within teams and together contribute to the improvement of health care delivery.[4]

Traditionally, medical students have added some value during clinical rotations to patient care directly rather than to health systems. The particularly helpful student might be a "team player" or an "outstanding student" but may not offer significant contributions to the clinical environment. As medical educators begin to recognize HSS as a crucial aspect of medical school curricula, they have begun to better articulate the skills involved and to create clear occasions for students to learn those skills. A number of medical schools around the US have created novel value-added roles for their students—as health coaches, patient navigators, care coordinators, quality improvement team extenders, or population health managers.[11] These programs leverage opportunities for students to improve the health of patients and populations while learning the core principles of HSS.[10,12] These emerging value-added roles represent the cumulative effort of medical educators, health system leaders, and community stakeholders working together to better integrate students into the health care team. Learners taking on these roles can make meaningful, recognizable contributions to care starting early in undergraduate medical education and spanning into graduate medical education.[8]

HISTORICAL VALUE-ADDED ROLES

In decades past, students often took on roles as valued clinical team members, performing tasks such as documentation, phlebotomy, and dressing changes, which arguably augmented their educational experience.[13] Since the 1990s, however, there has been a steady decline in the involvement of students in such roles. In many medical schools today, both preclerkship and clerkship students enter clinical sites largely as observers linked with attending physicians. At these sites, they are charged with learning "doctoring skills" such as the history and physical exam, key aspects of the doctor-patient relationship, and professionalism.[14] Over time, due to factors such as an increased focus on quality and expanded regulatory requirements, students have been offered fewer opportunities to document in the electronic health record (EHR) or to provide authentic contributions to team functioning.[15,16] In addition, the prevailing physician-student model, often dubbed a "preceptorship," requires time for physicians to educate and mentor students, which can decrease clinical efficiency and negatively impact productivity.[17,18] In these scenarios, student work can be relegated to the periphery, playing a nonessential role on health care teams.

There are different approaches to enhance learning for students, usually involving service-learning projects or team-based quality improvement endeavors, which have demonstrated some improved outcomes for learners and

TABLE 2.1	Historical Value-Added Roles for Medical Students			
Learning Roles	**Leaders and Potential Teachers/ Mentors**	**Context for Learning Experience**	**Operationalized Knowledge Domains**	**Opportunities for Further Value-Added Contributions**
Clinical preceptorships	Primarily physicians; also nurses, pharmacists, therapists, and patients	Clinical settings, including hospitals and primary care and specialty clinics	Patient care, knowledge for practice	• Observing supervisors • Practicing history-taking, physical examination, and communication skills • Perceived value added to health system by trainee and educational presence
Service-learning experiences	Community leaders and potentially families and patients	Community-based settings, including food pantries, homeless shelters, and health fairs	Professionalism	• Completing community-based projects • Value added to community and society by learner work
Student-run free clinics	Primarily physicians; also nurses and patients	Independent clinic commonly affiliated with a not-for-profit organization	Patient care, knowledge for practice, systems-based practice	• Performing diagnostic and therapeutic tasks with supervision • Value added to underserved patients by learner work

primary care practices.[19–21] However, the limited implementation of these types of programs speaks to how infrequently learners are consciously woven into the composition and work of a health care team. More often, learners become valued once they are able to contribute to clinical decisions, such as a diagnostic or therapeutic plan. In the sections that follow, we review some common contemporary student roles with an eye toward the operationalized knowledge and skills domains, the opportunities for value-added contributions, and the particular learning experience context (Table 2.1).

Clinical Preceptorships

The most prevalent experiential role for students in medical school is the clinical preceptorship. Many medical schools expose students to taking a history, performing a physical exam, and practicing communication skills early in their training in clinical skills courses and preceptorships. Later in their training, in the traditional clinical years, students undergo clerkships as the main method for developing knowledge and skills in various specialty areas. Under appropriate supervision by attending physicians, students are offered more opportunities for hands-on experience.

While these clinical preceptorship and clerkship encounters may create opportunities for students to learn essential clinical skills, they provide limited value to the health system. Medical educators typically point to improved clinician recruitment and retention, higher-quality patient care, and the fulfillment of a professional duty to educate the next generation of physicians as the system value provided by the preceptorship experience.[3,22] Other researchers suggest that the preceptorship does not consistently add value even though upper-level students at times can make valuable contributions to care in today's clinical environment.[14] Within the traditional medical student trajectory through preceptorships and clerkships, students begin on the outskirts of health care teams. They slowly become active contributors over the course of their medical school experiences and into residency training. In order to become part of the team, students must undergo a lengthy developmental phase, often taking years to become full participants in team functions. Frequent rotations from one service or clerkship to another further limits development and compromises longitudinal relationships with teams, mentors, and patients.[23] In this model, it is rare for students to make a difference beyond reporting and documenting.

Students as Educators

Another common way medical schools offer select students enhanced opportunities for learning is to challenge those students to help educate their colleagues. Students might lead wellness and burnout prevention exercises or participate in teaching programs in associated allied professions schools. After completing a course or set of courses, faculty might ask students to assist in the review and redesign of preclinical curricula they have just experienced. A similar approach is to incorporate students as evaluators of educational programs and have them offer suggestions for continuous improvement. Many schools have established "near-peer" mentor programs in which upper-level students offer advice and guidance to lower-level students or have incorporated second-year students as teachers of first-year students in clinical skills courses. In clinical settings, the supervising resident or attending might ask a student to educate the rest of the team about a new technology, care process, or the latest guidelines. By citing evidence-based medicine, students can challenge their supervisors to be up-to-date. By showing a senior colleague a new app, they might introduce their teammates to current clinical decision support tools.[11] While these opportunities can be meaningful for both students and the health care team, they tend not to be structured or offered to all students.

Service-Learning Experiences

The 2020–2021 Liaison Committee on Medical Education (LCME) guiding document, "Function and Standards of a Medical School," highlights **service learning** as a necessary element of the medical school experience:

> *Standard 6.6. The faculty of a medical school ensure that the medical education program provides sufficient opportunities for, encourages, and supports medical student participation in service-learning and/or community service activities.*[24]

Even before it became an LCME standard, medical educators have used service learning for decades to provide needed services to local settings and to link students with community-based sites.[25,26] Primarily designed to foster a sense of social justice or civic responsibility, service-learning roles may include volunteering at food pantries, homeless shelters, health fairs, or other community-based programs. Within the framework of service learning/community-based education developed by Magzoub and colleagues, most of these experiences would be considered "community exposure training-focused programs." Such programs provide few opportunities to integrate with the community or to provide direct services as part of a clinical team.[27] As such, there is limited research describing the benefit of such experiences to patients. There are other service-learning approaches within the Magzoub taxonomy that do provide more robust student roles and learning opportunities. One example of a primary care–oriented, training-focused program is at Morehouse School of Medicine and involves an interdisciplinary family health course designed to enhance student learning in community-based health while also providing services to families.[28,29] Nevertheless, these more integrated experiences, with potential for ongoing benefit for both the learners and the communities served, are rare. Medical school service-learning programs are typically not embedded within the health care **community of practice** and practice environment. Notably, many programs begin by linking students with "the best learning experience," rather than focusing on the patients most in need, which limits impact on patient outcomes.[28] Service learning plays an important role in fostering altruism and professional values and can potentially add value to patient care. Yet these experiences typically are not designed for learning HSS, do not occur within a collaborative clinical practice setting, and may not include clinical science education.

Student-Run Free Clinics

At their best, some research suggests that student-run free clinics can improve patient care skills and foster professional identity formation. Many student-run free clinics help students develop their own sense of themselves as future physicians and improve their clinical skills while providing needed medical care to patients who are underserved or underinsured.[30] Free clinics can provide rich opportunities for learning HSS; however, in actual practice, the focus of these experiences tends to be primarily on clinical skills development.[31,32] Students have limited opportunities for immersion into the local health system and with interprofessional partners, as these clinics are not well integrated into current day health systems. Most clinics are not scalable to host large numbers of students or patients. According to best estimates, less than 50% of medical schools have affiliated student-run free clinics and those that do cannot accommodate all students in longitudinal and immersive experiences in the clinic.[30,31] Finally, some authors have raised the ethical and moral issues involved when students perform higher-stakes clinical activities with vulnerable patient populations and have questioned the degree of supervision in these settings.[33]

Research and Systems Projects

One more way medical schools commonly involve students in enhanced roles with the potential to affect individual and population health is in health services research or health systems projects. Many of these approaches fall under a structured research requirement for students.

Students might perform basic or clinical science research that addresses local and broader needs for new knowledge or improved care delivery. Other approaches fall under a quality improvement elective for senior medical students. In these scenarios, students might do workflow or systems analysis, looking to identify "blind spots" in care delivery or points of care where physicians and other health care professionals could perform needed duties more efficiently. Finally, some medical schools with more of a community focus enlist students in community-based needs assessments to better understand the challenges of their local environment.[11] While all of these experiences do introduce students to crucial elements of HSS and have the potential to improve health outcomes, they often exist as episodic stand-alone projects. Students are not fully integrated into a local health care team or setting, and their work is more likely to be allocated to the periphery of core health care or health systems operations.

EMERGING VALUE-ADDED ROLES

Some versions of the models described earlier have existed unchanged for decades even though there have been notable changes in stated educational goals and in the culture of clinical settings. Two critical problems arise in maintaining current student experiences alongside a physician-centric professional development pathway. First, this pathway encourages the development of a "sovereign physician" professional identity that is at odds with interprofessional practice.[5] Second, students typically have minimal opportunity to become legitimate members of the practice team. The acculturation of the student into the health care system and the transition from learner to "physician contributor" is very slow. This educational model can seem outdated and in need of modification. The challenge for medical educators is increasingly clear: How can we help learners become valued members of a practice community while also acquiring knowledge, skills, and attitudes useful in a changing health system?[34]

In response to this challenge, a growing number of educators have started working with the premise that students can be embedded within health care's evolving interprofessional practice models while adding value, even from very early in their medical education.[12] These educators recognize that medical students are intrinsically motivated, academically talented, have a range of life experiences, and, had they not chosen to go to medical school, would be highly sought after by employers. These educators advocate for value-added medical education, as outlined in Chapter 1.[1,6,35,36] Ideally, value-added medical education entails both legitimate learning experiences that can add value and capacity to the health care system and can add

Students as Community and Population Health Managers: The A.T. Still University's School of Osteopathic Medicine in Arizona Example

Since unveiling its new curriculum on its Mesa, Arizona campus in 2012, the A.T. Still University's School of Osteopathic Medicine in Arizona (ATSU-SOMA) has continued to grow its unique "1 + 3" brand of value-added medical education. All students at ATSU-SOMA spend their first year in Arizona, but in partnership with the National Association of Community Health Centers, they embed themselves in 12 urban and rural community health centers across the country during the last 3 years of medical school. Students live in the communities they serve and work with local providers dedicated to serving underserved patients. This immersed experience allows learners to develop a fuller perspective of the challenges that patients face while trying to access health care services. Each of the 12 community campuses has dedicated classroom space for didactic sessions, clinical skills training, and instruction reinforcing osteopathic principles and practice. As community health centers, the sites provide care to a wide range of vulnerable populations. Students join health care teams serving patients with HIV, the urban homeless, recent immigrants, Native Americans, rural farmers in Appalachia, and Hawaiian natives. Using population health approaches and built upon a community-oriented primary care framework, students also have opportunities to develop and complete a community health project. The approach begins with identifying needs, moves to evaluating the identified need, and then involves implementing strategies for change. At a national conference for community health centers, participating students then compete for the honor of presenting their community projects.[43] See Chapter 10 for more information about this program.

value to the students' educational endeavors. Borrowing the definition proposed by Jed Gonzalo and colleagues at Penn State Hershey Medical Center, we contend that: Value-added medical education involves experiential roles for students in practice environments that have the potential to positively impact individual patient and population health outcomes, costs of care, or other processes within the health system while also enhancing student knowledge, attitudes, and skills in the clinical or health systems sciences.[37]

These emerging models recognize the compelling reasons for medical schools to develop and implement educational programs that serve their students and their local health care environments. The newer forms of value-added roles, detailed throughout this volume, have emerged out of different necessities. Implementing these models in a more widespread fashion has the potential to reinvigorate contemporary medical education by providing today's learners with the capabilities they will need in a dynamic health care system. Today's physician is no longer expected to have knowledge only of basic and clinical sciences but also to attain competencies in HSS. The core competencies embraced by HSS include population and public health; value-based care; quality improvement; health care structures and processes; health care policy, economics, and management; and clinical informatics and health information technology.[10] These competencies are often under-appreciated, but they encompass many aspects of community health and acknowledge the complex ways in which patients' lives are affected when interacting with the health care system. Value-added roles for students allow them opportunities to contribute to the patient's health care experience while they themselves learn about the system.

The sample programs that we highlight in text boxes in this chapter share some common features. To varying degrees, all involve patient-centered, interprofessional, team-based care models. Such models allow learners to transition from the periphery to a more proximal zone of patient care and activity within a health care setting. In addition, these programs place patients at the center, with a variety of physicians and other health care professionals with multiple complementary skills and areas of expertise providing care. The value-added clinical systems learning roles, meanwhile, allow students to immediately enter an interprofessional community that focuses on the overall needs of the patient and to simultaneously learn about both medicine and systems of care.[38,39] By experiencing interprofessional collaboration outside the classroom or simulation activities, students relate to physicians and other professionals on the team as contributors rather than as apprentices. Students are integral to the functioning of the team and enhance team performance, as opposed to being a burden for a supervising physician. For many of these programs, students also acquire new knowledge and skills in environments similar to those where they will one day practice as physicians.

So, what kinds of emerging value-added roles are students assuming early in medical school? This book showcases a number of examples, including serving as patient navigators, care coordinators, health coaches, and quality improvement team members.[8,40,41] Students can and do contribute to current health system needs, with appropriate support and oversight, by providing services not typically offered in certain settings. By way of illustration, students can serve as navigators, provide education or psychological or emotional support to patients, or facilitate access to care or community resources. Such work can lead to reduced readmissions, improved care transitions, and better patient self-care and satisfaction.[42] The skills that students attain in these roles accompany them as they progress into clerkships. Newly empowered, they can use these acquired skills to continue making meaningful contributions to patients and care teams while focusing on developing their clinical skills (Table 2.2). We highlight exemplar programs in text boxes scattered throughout this chapter.

PRIORITY AREAS FOR ADVANCING VALUE-ADDED ROLES AND PROGRAMS

Two years after implementing the patient navigator program, SyNC, the team at Penn State College of Medicine conducted a comprehensive review of the program. They performed on-site observations at 32 different clinical settings where their value-added roles curriculum was being carried out, conducted 29 one-on-one interviews with faculty, and held 4 student focus groups. Qualitative analysis of the review revealed important strategies for implementing such a program, themes for consideration when running such a program, and key features of the successful

---

Students as Care Coordinators: The Case Western Reserve University School of Medicine Example

In 2016, the Case Western Reserve University (CWRU) School of Medicine launched its value-added medical education program, based on the Penn State patient navigator approach. CWRU modified the Penn State model to focus more on care coordination and to target specific local populations. Placing students in two high-performing patient-centered medical homes—the VA Center of Excellence in Primary Care Education, which serves veterans, and Neighborhood Family Practice, a federally qualified community health center that serves primarily newly arrived refugee families—they become parts of established interprofessional teams. Each team manages and assesses the needs of a 20-patient panel within the practice. The student care coordinators perform a variety of functions on the health care team; program evaluations reveal positive impacts on the team and on patients as well as increased health systems knowledge for the students. The didactic curriculum includes trainings on the use of EHRs and registries for population health management, applied to specific populations.[43] More information about this program is in Chapter 5.

TABLE 2.2   Emerging Value-Added Roles for Medical Students

Role	Description	Potential Tasks
Patient navigators, health coaches, or "hot-spotters"	Students can be linked with clinical sites/programs to work with patients to achieve better outcomes, thereby extending the resources of the program. Patients can be identified by numerous mechanisms, including patients who are super-utilizers of care, those with complex medical conditions, or those in need of targeted interventions.	Acquiring an in-depth history to identify challenges/barriers to care, assessing health literacy, performing home visits to assess safety, accompanying patients to appointments, performing motivational interviewing, educating patients about disease processes or care plans, assessing adherence, and helping facilitate patient access to health portals, specialist providers, transportation, and community resources.
Care transitions facilitators	Students can be linked with clinical sites/programs that focus on the transition between settings, such as hospital and primary care clinic transition. Patients can be identified by readmission rates or those believed to be vulnerable during the transition.	In-depth interviewing with patients prior to the transition to review care plans, assess home situation and patient understanding, and help coordinate transportation and follow-up appointments. Following the transition, tasks can include phone calls to review care plans and ensure awareness of need for follow-up.
Safety and patient care analysts	Students can be integrated into health system processes by following a patient's course through the hospital or ambulatory care setting. Patients can be identified by preselected risk factors or from a convenience sample.	Analyzing the patient experience or process, identifying insufficiencies or vulnerable points in the continuum, and reporting results using the appropriate mechanism. Students can continue engaging with patients after they are discharged through phone calls or home visits. These activities can identify any medical errors or systems failures that were experienced by the patient. Students can report findings to hospital teams and initiate conversations about findings.
Quality improvement team extenders	Students can be integrated into quality improvement teams throughout health systems. Projects can be identified by anticipated duration, degree of complexity, and when aligned with students' available time.	Authentic contributions to the project team, including clinical assessments of the issue, interviews with key stakeholders, observations of clinical processes, collection of data, analysis, and presentation.
Population health managers	Students can be integrated into care teams to create physician-based or clinic-based patient registries stratified by disease process/clinical variable and identify gaps in care for the population of patients. Patient populations can be identified by quality metrics such as results of laboratory tests.	Using data analytics, operationalizing screening tools with patients or the population of patients, geo-mapping of resources/services, performing community or clinic-based needs assessments, designing or working on quality improvement project teams.
Patient care technicians or medication reconciliation assistants	Students can be trained to perform the tasks of a patient care technician and integrated into care teams in both ambulatory and hospital-based settings.	Performing intake assessments, acquiring vital signs, and assisting in triage duties. An extension of these roles could include medication reconciliation with patients during the intake process.
Medical scribes	Students can be trained to perform scribing activities and linked with provider-based teams in ambulatory and hospital-based settings to extend the work of providers.	Note taking and scribing of provider–patient encounters.

operation of value-added medical education. The crucial strategies identified for implementing value-added roles included thoughtful consideration of the following: student educational goals, patient characteristics, patient selection methods, activities to be performed, and resources. Those clinical sites with the most successful execution of the program, from the perspective of both administrators and faculty, shared five key features. First, they integrated students into interprofessional care teams to allow for interaction with work and processes. Second, they ensured that students were aware of the specific functions of the site and the student role within team. Third, they provided students the opportunity to be active, value-added participants in the clinical site rather than just observers. Fourth, they offered students the opportunity to have a high degree of continuity within the clinical site and with patients. Fifth, they developed a proactive continuous quality improvement process with regard to curriculum, student experience, and mentor experience. The review concluded that the overriding themes for consideration when contemplating a value-added clinical roles approach are (1) the value added to patient care from student work; (2) the educational benefit; (3) student engagement; (4) the working relationship between school, site, and students; (5) mentor time and site capacity; and (6) students' continuity at the site.[43] We review these six priority areas here in the form of questions medical educators might ask themselves when designing, implementing, or managing a value-added medical education endeavor.

How Might the New Student Roles Add Value Within Your Institution and/or Health System?

For a program to be successful, students and clinical partners should be able to recognize the ways that students can learn while providing a valuable service to patients or clients. As much as possible, the architects and managers of value-added medical education should investigate important potential activities and roles that students could play within or alongside the current activities and roles of other team members. How might students extend the work of any potential site and add value to patient care? These roles might be outside historical student roles; we encourage program developers and administrators to explore a wide range of possibilities. For example, students might be able to provide psychosocial support to patients, lighten the workload of care teams, or offer a "fresh pair of eyes" on a current process. They might add value by identifying community resources, providing education, and addressing patient barriers. We also recommend consulting with mentors who are invigorated by working with students who might be able to share teaching best practices. By contrast,

Students as Interprofessional Service-Learning Care Managers: The Florida International University Herbert Wertheim College of Medicine Example

Florida International University (FIU) Herbert Wertheim College of Medicine (HWCOM) launched the Green Family Foundation Neighborhood Health Education Learning Program (NeighborhoodHELP) in 2009. The longitudinal program involves 2 years of didactics introducing first- and second-year students to the social determinants of health (SDOH) and 3 years of household visits in underserved communities—for second-, third-, and fourth-year students. Supporting the program is a team of outreach workers who maintain relationships with households enrolled in the program and over 160 community providers. The medical school also runs mobile health centers (MHCs) for the delivery of integrated primary and behavioral health services and mammography screenings for participating household members. The MHCs provide care to uninsured and underinsured household members. For the home visits, each student is assigned to an interprofessional team from nursing, social work, and/or physician assistant studies; the teams are, in turn, assigned to an underserved household. Students act as health educators, health coaches, and care managers for household members while learning cultural humility, interprofessional collaboration, and practical skills related to motivational interviewing and the SDOH. Faculty from the medical school, as well as from partner health professions schools at FIU, participate in the home visits. Law and education faculty and students are available by referral. Students learn health systems science principles under the rubric of what the program calls "household-centered care": identifying and managing the SDOH that can improve the health outcomes for household members. After the first 2 years of the program, household surveys indicated that homes receiving student team visits reported increased use of preventive health services and decreased use of the emergency department. After 6 years of the program, compared with peers from other schools, graduating medical students reported more experience with clinical interprofessional education and addressing health disparities.[43] More information about this program is in Chapter 7.

at sites where mostly shadowing occurs, neither students nor mentors tend to find the program to be useful. Another important consideration when it comes to student roles is managing expectations. When embarking on a new clinical experience, there can often be disconnects between student expectations of what they should be doing and the work they actually perform. Some students hope to "save lives," and it takes effort to help students see the value of educating patients or identifying community-based resources.

What Particular Learning Goals Would the New Program Achieve for Students? What Gaps in Your Curriculum Might These New Roles Fill?

In addition to exploring the value added to the health system or local clinical environment, we advocate for thoughtful consideration of the value added to the students' learning experiences. Some of the learning goals may be available in historical and emerging value-added roles. Early exposure to patient care can help advance students' problem-solving skills, prepare them to recognize barriers that have impacts on patient health, and raise awareness of the time and resources required to effectively resolve a problem. Documenting in the EHR, perhaps as a scribe, can allow students to further develop informatics and information technology skills. Typically, mentors and students share the belief that these experiences could provide essential skills for future physicians. Some of the additional learning goals available with emerging value-added roles, associated with HSS, may require more consideration and care, as these goals depend on the details of the experience offered. Independent tasks—such as home visits, follow-up telephone calls, identification of community-based resources, and assisting patients in overcoming barriers—can offer opportunities to learn HSS skills such as practice management, insight into the insurance process, and teamwork. These goals, though, tend to materialize only when students are genuinely integrated into team processes and assigned autonomous tasks. In such scenarios, students and mentors report higher satisfaction and a higher likelihood of sustaining a value-added medical education endeavor. By contrast, situations in which students primarily shadow providers, complete repetitive tasks, or have limited autonomy or engagement tend to limit the perceived educational benefit.

How Would You Ensure Student Engagement and Assess Students Within These New Roles?

Student engagement with the enterprise can be an influential factor in any value-added program's success. Fully engaged students are able to proactively problem solve, assist patients, and recognize the work they perform as learning opportunities. Limited or half-hearted student engagement, by contrast, can be a barrier to success. One strategy for increasing engagement involves making changes even before medical school begins. This can include changing the admissions process to recruit different types of students who are more experienced and interested in broader service roles or setting up pilot programs to specifically attract engaged students. Once a program has begun, some reasons for limited engagement by students include having difficulty understanding the applicability of the program to their future careers or feeling underqualified for a role. Other students may need encouragement or prompting to understand how to assist patients and overcome barriers. To improve the degree of engagement, students typically need training at the site. As much as possible, it helps to align experiences with student interests and skills and to focus on the patient-centered aspects of the program. Providing opportunities for students to teach faculty new skills can also increase buy-in, as can starting these programs early in medical school, when students are more available and open to new experiences. A primary reason why a value-added roles program could falter stems from mentors. When frustrated, the mentors may feel an increased workload when students demonstrate limited engagement or motivation to contribute to patient-centered activities.

One additional way to foster increased student engagement lies in the assessment tools used for the curriculum. Assessment can be a powerful tool to foster student engagement, involvement, and investment in an activity. The Stanford Center for Opportunity Policy in Education has conducted extensive research on assessment strategies that both students and faculty find engaging and that motivate learners to continue with a particular course or curriculum. Their work has determined that six key qualities help foster engagement: relevance, authenticity, autonomy, collaboration, higher-order thinking skills, and self-assessment. Even though their work primarily centers on high school and college education, their recommendations in each of these areas can be fruitful for medical educators. To help students see the *relevance*, make connections to students' lived experiences and interests or through personalization. Involve them in and assess them on tasks in a value-added program linked to skills that they will use as physicians. *Authenticity* can arise in the construction of the program itself if it truly immerses students in the real-world work of the clinical setting. Any assessments that emerge should emphasize real-world connections and require students to solve real-world problems. As mentioned earlier, integrating students into a team fosters the success of a value-added experience and assessing on teamwork and *collaboration* can facilitate that integration. As much as possible, provide opportunities for students to collaborate in pairs or small groups to increase involvement in the task at hand. To emphasize *higher-order thinking skills*, try to emphasize tasks involving analysis, interpretation, and manipulation of information to solve a problem rather than simple data recording or collection. When developing assessments, ensure that the tasks have multiple solutions or involve various solution strategies. To highlight *autonomy*, build in opportunities for students to make choices that are consistent with their interests. Consider a range of tasks with accompanying assessments from which students can choose. Finally, curricular developers might contemplate the use of *self-assessment*. Requiring students to explain or justify their approaches or complete reflection exercises can help them assess their own learning and their own development.[44]

How Might You Evaluate the Success of the Program With Regard to Different Stakeholders—for Students, Faculty and Staff, and the Local Health System?

Logistically, the relationship between the school, sites, and students requires ongoing collaboration, communication, and problem solving for programmatic development, oversight, and improvement. In particular, to evaluate program success, the school and its partner sites should recognize the need for ongoing sharing of ideas across program sites

---

Students as Patient Navigators: The Penn State College of Medicine Example

In August 2014, Penn State College of Medicine launched its patient navigator value-added medical education program, known as Systems Navigation Curriculum or SyNC. SyNC combines immersive experiences as patient navigators with a course on health systems science (HSS). The 9-month patient navigator experience places first-year students in a variety of clinical sites. These sites include nursing homes, primary care clinics, specialty care clinics, underserved free clinics, and transitional care programs. Student navigators educate patients, provide information, facilitate coordination among different community care providers, and offer emotional support. Other roles can vary, ranging from assisting in implementing new clinic initiatives to serving as extensions of the clinical staff to guiding patients through the complex elements of a local health system or process. The accompanying classroom activities focus on HSS, and students must apply their patient navigator experiences to the lessons at hand. They are tasked with creating health care system improvement plans, personal reflections, and patient narratives. Their narratives and reflections focus on topics such as the changing composition of health care teams, the different roles played by different team members, including the evolving role of physicians, the perspectives of different stakeholders, and mindfulness.[43] More information about this program is in Chapter 4.

---

related to best practices. Different student-mentor pairings, different clinical teams, and different service sites can all communicate and collaborate to ensure the most optimal conditions for learning and patient care. It is also important to have mechanisms in place to evaluate both short- and long-term success. There might be challenges that needed to be addressed in the short term to achieve success in the long term. One critical recommendation involves the need for continuous improvement cycles. Putting in place such a quality improvement approach can help rapidly address problems and prevent future issues. One suggested approach would be to have monthly check-ins with core mentors and faculty and yearly "retreats" for a broader range of program participants, hosted by the school. These opportunities to get together can be vital for making improvements and for building a network between mentors. Similar to the processes related to student engagement, getting feedback and problem-solving input from students is critical. Students can help guide critical program improvements at the school level, including improving students' introduction to the program, setting up realistic expectations, and creating resources and guides. Successful value-added medical education programs rely on student and mentor feedback to continuously improve experiences.

What Resources Might a New Program Require, Including Faculty/Mentor Time, Curricular Time, Administrative Support, and Finances?
What Tools Might You Need to Determine Feasibility to Implement the Program?

When evaluating resources needed, it is important to consider faculty/mentor time, space within the curriculum, and any administrative and financial support needed. We focus in particular on faculty/mentor time and site capacity for student work, as these factors can be crucial for success. Mentor time can be particularly difficult to navigate. In general, students appreciate the educational benefit of working with mentors, but sometimes those same mentors can feel burdened. If the program is perceived as an "add-on" to the daily work of faculty or mentors, it can be difficult to launch or sustain. When designing a value-added roles program, it is crucial to strive to make the students' presence as burden-free as possible or contemplate ways in which mentors might receive time or support to complete extra tasks. Depending on the nature of the program, faculty or mentors could spend hours preparing for sessions and time during each session on patient selection and discussion of patient profiles with students. Strategizing about ways to recognize and reward participants for this time can help foster long-term success. Clinical space and resources can also be challenges, as a clinical site might have to locate empty desks or telephones for student use. If the program involves home visits or other efforts requiring drive time, it might be prudent to explore ways of compensating faculty or mentors for transportation costs. It also helps to be ready for changes at the clinical sites or partner facilities. Dynamic factors, such as the implementation of a new EHR, changes in staffing or funding, or structural changes at a location, can affect a site's ability to maintain participation in a program.

What Mechanisms Are Available to Foster Longitudinal Continuity for Students?

One critical feature of successful value-added clinical roles endeavors involves longitudinal continuity for students' work. That continuity can focus on mentors, sites, or patients—a combination of forms of continuity often works best.

Early Students as Clinical Microsystem Health Systems Improvement Partners: The University of California, San Francisco School of Medicine Example

The University of California, San Francisco (UCSF) School of Medicine launched its Bridges Curriculum in 2016. The program enables students to learn to work within complex systems as they contribute to improving health care outcomes. All first- and second-year medical students are placed within a longitudinal, interprofessional clinical microsystem at one of three health systems (academic, county, and veterans) in workplace learning communities led by physician coaches. In these longitudinal small groups, students learn professional behavior, apply clinical skills, and complete health systems improvement projects aligned with national and local priorities. Students start medical school with an immersion week within the assigned health system, learning about the patient experience, the patient population, and the interprofessional care delivery team. In the first few weeks, didactics and workshops offer the foundations of health systems science. Leveraging the structured Lean methodology soon after, student teams research the problem, determine project goals, conduct a gap analysis, implement interventions, and measure outcomes. At the end of 16 months, students present outcomes to deans and health system leaders, detailing their contributions to improving health care quality, value, safety and the patient experience. Since the implementation of the program, medical students have successfully contributed to hundreds of effective quality improvement initiatives in various medical disciplines and practice settings across multiple larger health systems.[43] See Chapter 8 for more information.

Even if students have specific assigned times during a week scheduled for a value-added experience, be prepared for events such as examinations, holidays, or other class events to disrupt regular participation. Such interruptions can hinder team integration and opportunities to contribute to patients and clinics as a whole. One possibility for improving continuity of care is to allow students the flexibility to follow up with patients or mentors outside of scheduled days.

CONCLUSION

With medical education and health systems undergoing significant transformation, we have reviewed some of the historical and emerging ways in which medical students have and can add value. Our hope is to provide perspective as medical schools learn to implement health systems science curricula successfully, including introducing experiential roles that fully immerse students into aspects of their local health care environments. We have reviewed some of the traditional ways in which students have added value and have highlighted exemplars of ways that medical schools across the US have begun to reimagine value-added roles for students. We have also delineated crucial areas for consideration and potential next steps for administrators thinking of initiating or revising a program focused on the value that medical education could contribute to patients and local health systems.

The potential ways in which students can add value are broad, ranging from point-of-care contributions to longitudinal patient outreach to quality improvement initiatives. We propose that educational and clinical value go hand in hand, and we challenge medical schools and clinical sites to work together to create experiences for students that achieve both goals. There are a range of strategies for enhancing educational value, including encouraging experiences outside of clinical sites, such as home visits, and ensuring that students receive feedback and assessments promoting engagement throughout the program. Meanwhile, students should be put in positions to provide value to the sites where they are assuming new roles. Interventions to foster student value include reframing student roles as "extenders" of clinic work and clinical care needs. Creating meaningful curricular space and priority for students to take advantage of opportunities for continuity with mentors and patients can help make these new extender roles successful. In order to maintain these successes, we recommend ongoing collaboration between schools and clinical sites to build shared goals and objectives. Working together, program partners can accommodate the inevitable disruptions and changes that will occur while developing a shared investment in education and patient outcomes.

We have identified facilitators, barriers, strategies, and best practices for implementing and maintaining value-added clinical systems learning roles. Understanding these elements is critical to sustaining community-based programs. Depending on the context, factors relating to students, including their engagement and perceived educational benefits, and those relating to partner sites, including the value added to clinical care, can be either facilitators or barriers to a program's success. By monitoring these factors, within a continuous quality improvement mindset, those responsible for a value-added medical education endeavor will be better prepared to sustain and grow the program. For students, it is essential to provide practical guides for the activities and assessments demanded, to make their roles as authentic as possible, and to allow opportunities for them to reflect and to see the relevance of the activities for their future careers. For mentors and faculty, attentiveness to time demands, students' schedules, clinical capacity, and space availability can play important roles in making the program rewarding and less burdensome. Building on historical roles and embracing emerging value-added learning roles can be key to addressing the challenge of educating systems-ready physicians of the future.

TAKE-HOME POINTS

1. Current health systems face pressures to transform at new levels unseen for decades. These pressures provide opportunities for medical educators, in partnership with their local health systems, to create value-added roles for their learners.
2. Medical schools have historically provided some value-added roles for students through experiences such as clinical preceptorships, service-learning experiences, and student-run free clinics.
3. Emerging value-added roles for students, which can provide richer experiential learning and exposure to health systems science, include possibilities such as patient navigation or coaching, care transition facilitation, safety and patient care analysis, quality improvement projects, and population health management.
4. The most successful value-added medical education programs thus far share some common features. They all involve patient-centered, interprofessional, team-based care models and place learners in a more proximal zone of patient care and activity within a health care setting.
5. Successful value-added roles embrace health systems science.
6. For a program to be successful, students and clinical partners should be able to recognize the ways that students can learn while providing a valuable service to patients or clients.

7. Successful programs honor the work of students on the team through learner assessments that reinforce important clinical and health systems science concepts.
8. When evaluating resources needed to establish value-added roles, it is important to consider faculty/mentor

---

Students as Quality Improvement Team Extenders: The University of North Carolina at Chapel Hill and the Vanderbilt University School of Medicine Examples

In 2016, the University of North Carolina School of Medicine launched its new value-added roles curriculum entitled "Translational Education at Carolina." This patient- and student-centered integrated program trains students to add value to the clinical care environment. Focusing on common clinical problems such as immunization rates, cancer screening, and diabetes care, students receive instruction in quality improvement techniques. The students then complete quality improvement projects in the clinics where they are training. Examples of successful projects include efforts to increase the percentage of diabetic patients who take a daily aspirin and to decrease the number of patients who fall away from care. The students design the projects, including setting the process and outcome measures, and the majority of the projects have had positive outcomes. Another successful project involved medical students teaching the proper documentation of diabetic foot exams in the EHR to other providers when the students noticed that the exams were often not being properly recorded. The project resulted in improved billing for diabetic foot exams and improved care for patients.[43] More information about this program is in Chapter 6.

Vanderbilt University School of Medicine has offered its own quality improvement (QI) curriculum, which has elements throughout all 4 years of medical school, since 2013. The longitudinal course, called "Foundations of Health Care Delivery," embeds students into care delivery systems for 4 years. First- and second-year students undergo a series of monthly seminars on health systems science topics, including patient safety and QI. Third- and fourth-year students complete further modules on patient safety and building a QI team and then direct their own QI projects. Illustrative projects include successful efforts to standardize the workflow of social work services in need-based clinics, to improve hand sanitation among health care workers, and to increase compliance with safety regulations related to the use of portable X-ray machines. All students must complete two plan-do-study-act (PDSA) cycles as part of their projects.[43] More information about this program is in Chapter 9.

time, space within the curriculum, any administrative and financial support needed, and the strength of the partnerships with local health systems.

QUESTIONS FOR FURTHER THOUGHT

1. What new student roles could add value within your institution and/or health system?
2. What particular learning goals could a new program achieve for students? What gaps in your curriculum might these new roles fill?
3. How would you ensure student engagement and assess students within these new roles?
4. How might you evaluate the success of a new program on different stakeholders—for students, faculty and staff, and the local health system?
5. What resources might a new program require, including faculty/mentor time, curricular time, administrative support, and finances?

ANNOTATED BIBLIOGRAPHY

Dornan T, Boshuizen H, King N, Scherpbier A. Experience-based learning: a model linking the processes and outcomes of medical students' workplace learning. *Med Educ.* 2007;41(1):84–91. https://doi.org/10.1111/j.1365-2929.2006.02652.x.
This seminal article highlights the ways in which opportunities for authentic experiential learning in medical education have changed over time. The authors provide a model for effective workplace learning and advocate for what they call "supported participation," in which students gain practical competence while being given the assistance and resources needed to acquire confidence, motivation, and a sense of professional identity.

Gonzalo JD, Thompson BM, Haidet P, Mann K, Wolpaw DR. A constructive reframing of student roles and systems learning in medical education using a communities of practice lens. *Acad Med.* 2017;92(12):1687–1694. https://doi.org/10.1097/ACM.0000000000001778.
Using key features of community-of-practice theory, the authors contrast current and new experiential learning roles for medical students. They propose the concept of "value-added clinical systems learning roles" as a way to provide students with opportunities to make meaningful contributions to patient care while learning health systems science at the patient and population level.

Gonzalo JD, Dekhtyar M, Hawkins RE, Wolpaw DR. How can medical students add value? Identifying roles, barriers, and strategies to advance the value of undergraduate medical education to patient care and the health system. *Acad Med.* 2017;92(9):1294–1301. https://doi.org/10.1097/ACM.0000000000001662.
This article summarizes takeaways from a 2016 American Medical Association Accelerating Change in Medical Education conference, in which participants met to explore value-added medical education. The conference of educators, AMA staff, students, and systems leaders identified potential new learning roles for students and noted six priority areas for advancing value-added medical education.

Gonzalo JD, Graaf D, Johannes B, Blatt B, Wolpaw DR. Adding value to the health care system: identifying value-added systems roles for medical students. *Am J Med Qual.* 2017;32(3):261–270. https://doi.org/10.1177/1062860616645401.
This study provides the results of a 2-year investigation. The investigators toured multiple clinical sites and interviewed stakeholders for their perceptions and ideas with regard to enhanced systems roles for students at their sites. Thematic analysis revealed potential new categories of new systems roles, anticipated benefits for clinics and students, and the elements of a framework for value-added student roles.

Gonzalo JD, Graaf D, Ahluwalia A, Wolpaw DR, Thompson BM. A practical guide for implementing and maintaining value-added clinical systems learning roles for medical students using a diffusion of innovations framework. *Adv Health Sci Educ.* 2018;23(4):699–720. https://doi.org/10.1007/s10459-018-9822-5.
Utilizing a diffusions-of-innovations framework, the authors explore and identify barriers, facilitators, and best practices for implementing value-added clinical systems learning roles for medical students. They identified six important factors that influence program implementation and maintenance, including educational benefit, value added to patient care, student engagement, and mentor time and site capacity.

REFERENCES

1. Grumbach K, Lucey CR, Johnston SC. Transforming from centers of learning to learning health systems: the challenge for academic health centers. *JAMA.* 2014;311(11):1109. https://doi.org/10.1001/jama.2014.705.
2. Berwick DM, Nolan TW, Whittington J. The Triple Aim: care, health, and cost. *Health Aff (Millwood).* 2008;27(3):759–769. https://doi.org/10.1377/hlthaff.27.3.759.
3. Ogrinc GS, Headrick LA, Boex JR. Understanding the value added to clinical care by educational activities. Value of Education Research Group. *Acad Med.* 1999;74(10):1080–1086. https://doi.org/10.1097/00001888-199910000-00009.
4. Smith MD, Institute of Medicine (US) eds. *Best Care at Lower Cost: The Path to Continuously Learning Health Care in America.* Washington, DC: National Academies Press; 2013.
5. Lucey CR. Medical education: part of the problem and part of the solution. *JAMA Intern Med.* 2013;173(17):1639. https://doi.org/10.1001/jamainternmed.2013.9074.
6. Sklar DP. How medical education can add value to the health care delivery system. *Acad Med.* 2016;91(4):445–447. https://doi.org/10.1097/ACM.0000000000001103.
7. Ehrenfeld JM, Spickard WA, Cutrer WB. Medical student contributions in the workplace: can we put a value on priceless? *J Med Syst.* 2016;40(5). https://doi.org/10.1007/s10916-016-0494-5.

8. Gonzalo JD, Graaf D, Johannes B, Blatt B, Wolpaw DR. Adding value to the health care system: identifying value-added systems roles for medical students. *Am J Med Qual.* 2017;32(3):261–270. https://doi.org/10.1177/1062860616645401.

9. Weiss KB, Bagian JP, Nasca TJ. The clinical learning environment: the foundation of graduate medical education. *JAMA.* 2013;309(16):1687. https://doi.org/10.1001/jama.2013.1931.

10. Gonzalo JD, Dekhtyar M, Starr SR, et al. Health systems science curricula in undergraduate medical education: identifying and defining a potential curricular framework. *Acad Med.* 2017;92(1):123–131. https://doi.org/10.1097/ACM.0000000000001177.

11. Gonzalo JD, Dekhtyar M, Hawkins RE, Wolpaw DR. How can medical students add value? Identifying roles, barriers, and strategies to advance the value of undergraduate medical education to patient care and the health system. *Acad Med.* 2017;92(9):1294–1301. https://doi.org/10.1097/ACM.0000000000001662.

12. Gonzalo JD, Haidet P, Papp KK, et al. Educating for the 21st-century health care system: an interdependent framework of basic, clinical, and systems sciences. *Acad Med.* 2017;92(1).35–39. https://doi.org/10.1097/ACM.0000000000000951.

13. Ludmerer KM. *Time to Heal: American Medical Education from the Turn of the Century.* New York: Oxford University Press; 2005.

14. Dornan T, Boshuizen H, King N, Scherpbier A. Experience-based learning: a model linking the processes and outcomes of medical students' workplace learning. *Med Educ.* 2007;41(1):84–91. https://doi.org/10.1111/j.1365-2929.2006.02652.x.

15. Kuhn T, Basch P, Barr M, Yackel T. Clinical documentation in the 21st century: executive summary of a policy position paper from the American College of Physicians. *Ann Intern Med.* 2015;162(4):301. https://doi.org/10.7326/M14-2128.

16. Gonzalo JD, Baxley E, Borkan J, et al. Priority areas and potential solutions for successful integration and sustainment of health systems science in undergraduate medical education. *Acad Med.* 2017;92(1):63–69. https://doi.org/10.1097/ACM.0000000000001249.

17. Shea S, Nickerson K, Tenenbaum J, et al. Compensation to a department of medicine and its faculty members for the teaching of medical students and house staff. *Am J Ophthalmol.* 1996;121(4):469. https://doi.org/10.1016/S0002-9394(14)70474-X.

18. Christner JG, Dallaghan GB, Briscoe G, et al. The community preceptor crisis: recruiting and retaining community-based faculty to teach medical students—a shared perspective from the Alliance for Clinical Education. *Teach Learn Med.* 2016;28(3):329–336. https://doi.org/10.1080/10401334.2016.1152899.

19. Henschen BL, Bierman JA, Wayne DB, et al. Four-year educational and patient care outcomes of a team-based primary care longitudinal clerkship. *Acad Med.* 2015;90(11 suppl):S43–S49. https://doi.org/10.1097/ACM.0000000000000897.

20. Gould BE, Grey MR, Huntington CG, et al. Improving patient care outcomes by teaching quality improvement to medical students in community-based practices. *Acad Med.* 2002;77(10):1011–1018. https://doi.org/10.1097/00001888-200210000-00014.

21. Olney CA, Livingston JE, Fisch SI, Talamantes MA. Becoming better health care providers: outcomes of a primary care service-learning project in medical school. *J Prev Inter Community.* 2006;32(1-2):133–147. https://doi.org/10.1300/J005v32n01_09.

22. Veloski J. The value added to clinical care by medical education. *Health Policy Newsletter.* 1998;11(2):Article 5. https://core.ac.uk/download/pdf/46969067.pdf. Published online January 1, 2005. Accessed 15.04.21.

23. Hirsh DA, Ogur B, Thibault GE, Cox M. "Continuity" as an organizing principle for clinical education reform. *N Engl J Med.* 2007;356(8):858–866. https://doi.org/10.1056/NEJMsb061660.

24. Liaison Committee on Medical Education. Functions and Structures of a Medical School 2020–2021. https://medicine.mercer.edu/wp-content/uploads/sites/7/2020/01/2020-21_Functions-and-Structure_2019-10-04-1-1.pdf. Published online March 2019. Accessed 26.05.21.

25. Clayton PH, Bringle RG, Hatcher JA, eds. Research on Service Learning: Conceptual Frameworks and Assessment: Communities, Institutions, and Partnerships. *Stylus Pub*; 2013.

26. Hunt JB, Bonham C, Jones L. Understanding the goals of service learning and community-based medical education: a systematic review. *Acad Med.* 2011;86(2):246–251. https://doi.org/10.1097/ACM.0b013e3182046481.

27. Magzoub MEMA, Schmidt HG. A taxonomy of community-based medical education. *Acad Med.* 2000;75(7):699–707. https://doi.org/10.1097/00001888-200007000-00011.

28. Davidson RA, Waddell R. A historical overview of interdisciplinary family health: a community-based interprofessional health professions course. *Acad Med.* 2005;80(4):334–338. https://doi.org/10.1097/00001888-200504000-00005.

29. Buckner AV, Ndjakani YD, Banks B, Blumenthal DS. Using service-learning to teach community health: the Morehouse School of Medicine Community Health Course. *Acad Med.* 2010;85(10):1645–1651. https://doi.org/10.1097/ACM.0b013e3181f08348.

30. Simpson SA, Long JA. Medical student-run health clinics: important contributors to patient care and medical education. *J Gen Intern Med.* 2007;22(3):352–356. https://doi.org/10.1007/s11606-006-0073-4.

31. Chen HC, Sheu L, O'Sullivan P, ten Cate O, Teherani A. Legitimate workplace roles and activities for early learners. *Med Educ.* 2014;48(2):136–145. https://doi.org/10.1111/medu.12316.

32. Meah YS, Smith EL, Thomas DC. Student-run health clinic: novel arena to educate medical students on systems-based practice. *Mt Sinai J Med.* 2009;76(4):344–356. https://doi.org/10.1002/msj.20128.

33. Buchanan D, Witlen R. Balancing service and education: ethical management of student-run clinics. *J Health*

Care Poor Underserved. 2006;17(3):477–485. https://doi.org/10.1353/hpu.2006.0101.

34. Jonassen DH, Land SM, eds. *Theoretical Foundations of Learning Environments*. Mahwah, NJ: L. Erlbaum Associates; 2000.

35. Curry RH. Meaningful roles for medical students in the provision of longitudinal patient care. *JAMA*. 2014;312(22):2335. https://doi.org/10.1001/jama.2014.16541.

36. Lin SY, Schillinger E, Irby DM. Value-added medical education: engaging future doctors to transform health care delivery today. *J Gen Intern Med*. 2015;30(2):150–151. https://doi.org/10.1007/s11606-014-3018-3.

37. Gonzalo JD, Thompson BM, Haidet P, Mann K, Wolpaw DR. A constructive reframing of student roles and systems learning in medical education using a communities of practice lens. *Acad Med*. 2017;92(12):1687–1694. https://doi.org/10.1097/ACM.0000000000001778.

38. Zwarenstein M, Goldman J, Reeves S. Interprofessional collaboration: effects of practice-based interventions on professional practice and healthcare outcomes. In: *Cochrane Database of Systematic Reviews*. The Cochrane Collaboration. West Sussex, UK: John Wiley & Sons, Ltd; 2009. https://doi.org/10.1002/14651858.CD000072.pub2.

39. Reeves S, Pelone F, Harrison R, Goldman J, Zwarenstein M. *Interprofessional collaboration to improve professional practice and healthcare outcomes*. Cochrane Effective Practice and Organisation of Care Group, ed. *Cochrane Database of Systematic Reviews*. Published online June 22, 2017. https://www.cochranelibrary.com/cdsr/doi/10.1002/14651858.CD000072.pub3/full. Accessed 26.05.21.

40. Chang A, Ritchie C. Patient-centered models of care: closing the gaps in physician readiness. *J Gen Intern Med*. 2015;30(7):870–872. https://doi.org/10.1007/s11606-015-3282-x.

41. Onie RD. Creating a new model to help health care providers write prescriptions for health. *Health Aff (Millwood)*. 2012;31(12):2795–2796. https://doi.org/10.1377/hlthaff.2012.1116.

42. Freeman HP, Rodriguez RL. History and principles of patient navigation. *Cancer*. 2011;117(15 suppl):3539–3542. https://doi.org/10.1002/cncr.26262.

43. Gonzalo JD, Graaf D, Ahluwalia A, Wolpaw DR, Thompson BM. A practical guide for implementing and maintaining value-added clinical systems learning roles for medical students using a diffusion of innovations framework. *Adv Health Sci Educ*. 2018;23(4):699–720. https://doi.org/10.1007/s10459-018-9822-5.

44. Bae S, Kokka K. *Student Engagement in Assessments: What Students and Teachers Find Engaging*. Stanford, CA: Stanford Center for Opportunity Policy in Education; 2016.

The Role of Program Evaluation in Value-Added Medical Education: Overall Outcomes and Connections to the Assessment of Learning

Jamie Fairclough, Sally Santen, Leslie Sheu, and Judee Richardson

LEARNING OBJECTIVES

1. Describe the role and utility of program evaluation in value-added medical education.
2. Recall key questions to consider when developing a comprehensive evaluation plan.
3. Compare and contrast evaluation types, methods, and tools to capture and organize data that align with the evaluation plan.
4. Identify an evaluation framework that can be used to measure and assess achievement of learning outcomes for value-added educational activities.
5. Describe how program evaluation and assessment of learning are interconnected.
6. Explain why stakeholder engagement is an important aspect of program evaluation planning and implementation.

OUTLINE

CHAPTER SUMMARY

In this chapter, we provide a formal definition of program evaluation that is specific to medical education and discuss the importance of evaluation planning for value-added medical education programs. We then identify five types of evaluation and introduce various methods and tools that can be used to develop an evaluation plan, including the logic model. We describe how an evaluation framework can serve as a guide in the design of educational activities that demonstrate student achievement of targeted learning outcomes. We also describe how to align assessments with program objectives and elements of an evaluation. Finally, we explain why it is important to engage internal and external stakeholders throughout the evaluation process.

PROGRAM EVALUATION: UTILITY IN MEDICAL EDUCATION

A formal evaluation process is key to documenting outcomes for institutional stakeholders and improving the quality of education programs. Over the years, evaluation experts have expanded definitions and operationalized frameworks to guide evaluation efforts and activities. Among many evaluation definitions proposed, two are particularly noteworthy for medical educators. In its March 2018 document, entitled *Functions and Structure of a Medical School: Standards for Accreditation of Medical Education Programs Leading to the MD Degree*, the Liaison Committee on Medical Education (LCME) defined **evaluation** as "the systematic use of a variety of methods to collect, analyze, and use information to determine whether a program is fulfilling its mission(s) and achieving its goal(s)."[1] To help medical schools focus their evaluation efforts, the LCME developed a related accreditation standard and corresponding elements to guide medical education evaluation activities.

LCME Standard 8.4 (entitled, "Evaluation of Educational Program Outcomes") outlines expectations for evaluating the overall quality of medical education programs, which includes the assessment of any didactic and/or experiential activities that have the potential to impact student outcomes, patient care, and the health care delivery system.[1] Because the LCME accredits most US medical schools, educators around the country have a vested interest in developing or adopting new approaches and refining existing methods to improve evaluation data tracking and monitoring.

A second definition that is of importance to medical educators comes from the Centers for Disease Control and Prevention (CDC). The CDC defines evaluation as a systematic method for collecting, analyzing, and utilizing data to assess the effectiveness and efficiency of programs. To provide further guidance, the CDC adopted 30 standards from the Joint Committee on Standards for Educational Evaluation and organized them into four categories to assist organizations with the development of evaluation plans.[2] For the purposes of this chapter, we wanted to formulate a definition of evaluation that was specific to medical education. In doing so, we considered various aspects of LCME and CDC definitions and standards and resolved to formally define medical education evaluation as a systematic process involving the collection, analysis, and comparison of data against a set of standards or established criteria to assess quality, impact, and effectiveness of medical education programs.

In 2010, Vassar and colleagues published an article in the *Journal of Educational Evaluation for Health Professions* highlighting the utility of program evaluation in medical education. The authors asserted that systematic, utilization-focused evaluation procedures can assist institutions in answering questions about the overall quality and effectiveness of medical education programs and, consequently, value-added medical education activities.[3] As utilization-focused evaluations are considered to be beneficial only when so deemed by intended users of the findings, medical educators need to stay abreast of interests and expectations set forth by internal and external stakeholders. When external stakeholders include accrediting agencies (such as the LCME), we necessarily incorporate standards and thresholds that further demonstrate success and justify resource needs that are necessary to fulfill the institution's mission and achieve the goals of the program. When external stakeholders include public health institutions (such as the CDC), we need to ensure that the standards used, the metrics selected, and the thresholds established are appropriate for evaluating program quality and effectiveness.

Now that we have a broader understanding of program evaluation and its relevance to medical education, we will explore specific components of a comprehensive evaluation program. Subsequent sections of this chapter focus on the development of an evaluation plan for value-added programs; discussion of evaluation types, methods, and tools used in evaluation planning and implementation; description of an evaluation framework to estimate achievement of learning outcomes aligned with educational activities and assessment strategies; and considerations for stakeholder engagement in the evaluation process.

DEVELOPING AN EVALUATION PLAN

An **evaluation plan** is a living document that is best referred to throughout program development and implementation, data collection, data analysis, reporting, and recommendation stages. The plan can be viewed as a topographical map for the education team as they encounter ups and downs (mountains and valleys), unanticipated barriers (bodies of water, dams, elevation changes), and smooth progress (clear roads and pathways). It also helps the team to remain focused on the purpose of the evaluation, measurable goals, and how evidence-based success will be achieved. Thus, a high-quality and oft-referenced evaluation plan is essential.

A common and useful first step in developing an evaluation plan is to ask critical questions. For example: What are you trying to accomplish (i.e., what is your goal)? What and where are the gaps in the current environment? Is there a need to have those gaps filled? What is the best way to fill those gaps? What are the highest quality results, and what evidence do you need to attain them? How will you use the information gathered to inform decision-making and strategic planning?

The CDC recommends asking and clarifying three core questions in the evaluation plan[4]:

1. What is the program to be evaluated, and how are anticipated outcomes linked to the original objectives?
2. How will the program be designed and implemented? (This is often referred to as the process evaluation.)
3. Why is this program needed? What are the gaps in current knowledge and/or need that the program intends to fill?

The CDC also recommends engaging stakeholders early in the evaluation planning process and describing the program clearly in the evaluation plan itself.[4] It encourages focusing the evaluation design on what is feasible within time constraints, budgetary envelopes, political climate and acceptability, and quality assurance controls. Ongoing editing and reevaluation of various components of the plan is necessary.

In 1999, the CDC proposed a graphical representation of evaluation that is still widely used today (Fig. 3.1).[4,5] In the outer circle of the graphic, there are steps in the evaluation process that include engaging stakeholders, describing the program, focusing the evaluation design, gathering credible evidence, justifying conclusions drawn, ensuring use, and sharing lessons learned. These steps are not always linear because of the back-and-forth nature of planning

and implementation. It is important to take time with each step as the specific context and program are considered.

Moving inward to the next circle of the graphic, there are standards introduced for strong evaluation in public health. These standards are grouped within four areas: **utility**, **feasibility**, **propriety**, and **accuracy**,[5] all of which apply to every step and phase of the evaluation plan and its implementation. Utility refers to the way in which information collected will serve the needs of the intended users. Feasibility refers to maintaining a realistic, prudent, diplomatic, and frugal approach. Propriety includes legal and ethical behavior at all times, with regard for the welfare of those involved and those affected. Accuracy includes the comprehensiveness of the evaluation and its unwavering grounding in data.

In its book, *WHO Evaluation Practice Handbook*, the World Health Organization (WHO) made recommendations that aligned with the CDC's framework for evaluation planning and implementation, including focusing on the relationship between expected and achieved outcomes by examining the processes leading from one to the other (CDC question #2).[6] The organization also recommends focusing on the relevance, impact, effectiveness, efficiency, and sustainability of the interventions and their contributions (CDC questions, #1, #2, and #3). Finally, by providing

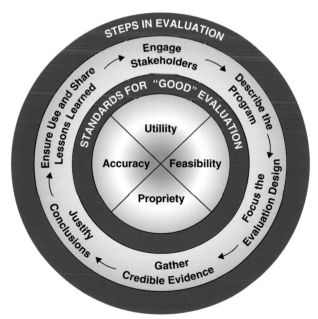

Fig. 3.1 Centers for Disease Control and Prevention Framework for Program Evaluation. (National Center for Chronic Disease Prevention and Health Promotion. *Developing an Effective Evaluation Plan: Setting the Course for Effective Program Evaluation.* Centers for Disease Control and Prevention. http://www.cdc.gov/obesity/downloads/CDC-Evaluation-Workbook-508.pdf. Published 2011. Accessed December 11, 2020.)

evidence-based information that is credible, reliable, and useful, evaluators will inform decision-making and strategic planning cycles of program development (CDC question #3).

In alignment with CDC and WHO recommendations, an evaluation plan should be thorough and holistic and should include research questions, methods, analyses, and a description of the intended usage/presentation of results. In developing the plan, it is important to remember to:

- Begin planning the evaluation early;
- Engage stakeholders early, clearly articulating the identified need, goals, and purpose;
- Select a high-quality, valid, and reliable methodological design and analytic plan;
- Pay attention to how results will be used and to whom and in what format they will be communicated; and
- Collect data of high quality and high utility.

The exact planning approach and specific steps to take will depend on the type of evaluation chosen and the specific methods and tools selected to capture and monitor data. Thus, educators need to identify these factors at the time when core questions are being asked and answered.

EVALUATION TYPES, METHODS, AND TOOLS

During the course of writing this chapter, the medical field found itself at the front lines of the COVID-19 pandemic. The Association of American Medical Colleges (AAMC) issued multiple guidance documents for medical schools related to student clinical participation (March 17, 2020), direct patient contact activities (March 30, 2020), and medical student roles (April 14, 2020). Subsequent release of an August 14, 2020 document replaced earlier guidance with updates regarding medical students' use of personal protective equipment and student participation in direct, in-person clinical care.[7] Given the dramatic and rapid changes to student roles in clinical settings, both because of limitations (e.g., for face-to-face activities with patients) as well as opportunities (e.g., for implementation projects), evaluation has proven essential to ensure ongoing adaptation of roles as local experiences, real-time scientific knowledge, and medical guidelines continued to evolve during COVID-19. Program developers have needed to remain updated on the health and safety concerns of COVID-19 and the potential impacts that AAMC recommendations have had on medical schools' evaluation and assesment efforts.

No matter the context, to choose the best evaluation type, method, and tools for a given program, we must first consider the evaluation goal. Early on in a program's development, the goal of evaluation may be to acquire feedback to ensure that a program or activity is feasible and appropriately connected to objectives. Over time, the evaluation

may switch to focus more on outcomes or impact. In Table 3.1, we compare formative, summative, process, outcomes, and impact evaluations and provide examples of how each can be used to specifically evaluate value-added medical education programs and COVID-19 projects.

Once an evaluation type is selected, the planning team needs to determine the best evaluation method that aligns with the program's outcomes. Quantitative, qualitative, or mixed methods can be used to capture various types of evaluation data for any planned approach (e.g., utilization-focused approach, objectives-oriented approach).[8,9]

- **Quantitative methods** provide numeric, countable data that can be used to measure outputs and quantify impact. Quantitative data can be collected from surveys, assessments, questionnaires, exams, rubrics, and other data collection instruments.
- **Qualitative methods** provide more nuanced and subjective data. These methods can be used to acquire information that answers questions regarding process, value, and accountability, some of which may be difficult to quantify. Qualitative measures answer questions that are open-ended rather than discrete; the data can be captured from observations, interviews, case studies, or focus groups. The value in capturing qualitative data is that it provides more detailed answers to probing questions, such as *Why? How? In what way? To what extent?*
- **Mixed methods** combine elements from both quantitative and qualitative approaches, which can be complementary to one another. Quantitative methods can provide information on questions requiring further insight than can be gained through qualitative methods. Conversely, qualitative methods can provide initial data to inform the design of quantitative surveys to administer to a broader audience.

Just as there are different methods that can inform evaluation planning, there are also different tools that can facilitate the collection of quantitative data and qualitative evidence that demonstrate program success. A **logic model** with guiding questions, in combination with an **evaluation plan**, can help shape an evaluation approach.

According to the WK Kellogg Foundation, a logic model is an action-oriented tool used for program evaluation and strategic reporting activities.[10] The CDC formally defines a logic model as "a graphic depiction (road map) that presents the shared relationships among the resources, activities, outputs, outcomes, and impact for your program."[11] When key elements of the program are captured and linearly displayed in a logic model, stakeholders can visualize the way in which various components and program activities align with expected outcomes. Although logic models vary based on the size and composition of

TABLE 3.1	Evaluation Types, Definitions, and Examples Related to the COVID-19 Pandemic	
Evaluation Type	Definition	Examples Specific to Value-Added Medical Education Programs
Formative evaluation	Evaluation of a program's value, often during the development of a program, with the goal of making early modifications to improve the program.	Frequent feedback from stakeholders (students, facilitators, systems leaders, education leaders) to ensure that goals are being met. COVID-19 Example: Obtain feedback from supervising faculty/residents on the perceived value students add while staffing COVID-19 testing sites/phone centers.
Summative evaluation	Evaluation at the end of a program (or part of the program) to understand its effectiveness.	Surveys or interviews of stakeholders upon completion of the first year of a value-added program with questions regarding the value of specific activities and whether learning objectives were met. Knowledge-based exams to assess whether learning objectives were met. COVID-19 Example: Evaluate the utility of a COVID-19 resource guide that was developed by medical students.
Process evaluation	Evaluation of specific activities to determine whether they were implemented as intended.	Surveys or focus groups at the end of activities that are linked to implementation strategies. Observations of activities to evaluate whether they were implemented as intended and to troubleshoot inefficiencies or misunderstandings. COVID-19 Example: Utilize a checklist to ensure that students properly document telehealth services provided.
Outcomes evaluation	Evaluation of changes in knowledge, attitudes, and behaviors as a result of the program.	Surveys, interviews, or focus groups for students, trainees, or patients on outcomes of their participation in the program (including knowledge, comfort, skills). COVID-19 Example: Interview health system leaders regarding their attitudes toward student engagement in COVID-19 quality improvement (QI) efforts.
Impact evaluation	Evaluation of long-term, sustained changes as a result of the program.	Review of student QI project outcomes over time and changes in health system flow or patient outcomes as a result of student engagement. COVID-19 Example: Assess the extent to which COVID-19 workflows are updated to reflect the value-added roles of medical students.

programs and the complexity of the evaluation process, both the WK Kellogg Foundation and the CDC recommend the use of a model that captures (at a minimum) program information pertaining to the following: (1) inputs, (2) activities, (3) outputs, (4) outcomes (which may be short term, intermediate, or long term), and (5) impacts. Definitions of these components[10,11] are provided here:

- **Inputs:** Resources used to implement a program; may include financial, physical, and/or human resources.
- **Activities:** Processes and/or actions used to implement a program.
- **Outputs:** Products of program activities.
- **Outcomes:** Results used to determine whether a program met its anticipated goals; can be short term, intermediate, or long term.
- **Impacts:** Measurable changes that occur as a result of program implementation.

Using a combination of methods, tools, and core questions can strengthen evaluation findings. Logic models containing vital pieces of information can help faculty develop insightful questions that can be used to guide planning efforts and shape the processes established to

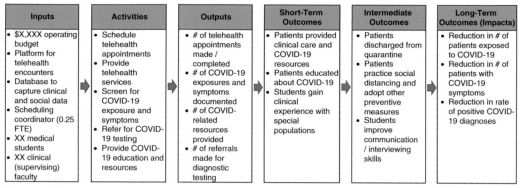

Inputs	Activities	Outputs	Short-Term Outcomes	Intermediate Outcomes	Long-Term Outcomes (Impacts)
• $X,XXX operating budget • Platform for telehealth encounters • Database to capture clinical and social data • Scheduling coordinator (0.25 FTE) • XX medical students • XX clinical (supervising) faculty	• Schedule telehealth appointments • Provide telehealth services • Screen for COVID-19 exposure and symptoms • Refer for COVID-19 testing • Provide COVID-19 education and resources	• # of telehealth appointments made / completed • # of COVID-19 exposures and symptoms documented • # of COVID-related resources provided • # of referrals made for diagnostic testing	• Patients provided clinical care and COVID-19 resources • Patients educated about COVID-19 • Students gain clinical experience with special populations	• Patients discharged from quarantine • Patients practice social distancing and adopt other preventive measures • Students improve communication / interviewing skills	• Reduction in # of patients exposed to COVID-19 • Reduction in # of patients with COVID-19 symptoms • Reduction in rate of positive COVID-19 diagnoses

Fig. 3.2 Sample Logic Model. Project: Student-Delivered Telehealth Services for Indigent Patients Under Quarantine for COVID-19.

evaluate the quality and success of value-added medical education programs. Once all questions are developed, it is helpful to map those questions back to the logic model. This mapping can help leaders identify the following early on in the process: (1) aspects of the program that will be evaluated, (2) the program activities that are most related to outcomes of interest, (3) data collection methods and data reporting needs, and (4) implementation procedures and timelines. Because all relevant details are included in a logic model, program developers can more readily determine the degree to which their program was implemented as planned and identify the quantifiable outputs that were produced as a direct result of related activities. They can also assess whether the program's short-term, intermediate, and long-term outcomes were achieved, given available resources and assumptions. Asking relevant questions that take stakeholder expectations, interests, and needs into consideration can help medical schools prioritize evaluation activities and focus evaluation methods on those that are most essential for operations and reporting. Other questions that may not be added to the logic model but still should be considered include the following[11]:

1. What is the target audience for each aspect of the program?
2. What questions will the target audience have about the program (as it relates to their own interests and reporting needs)?
3. How will the target audience use the information that is obtained from a formal evaluation process?

To further illustrate the feasibility of the logic model as an effective tool for evaluating value-added medical education, a sample model based on a new value-added student program during COVID-19 is provided (Fig. 3.2).

THE EVALUATION FRAMEWORK

A rigorous program evaluation will start with program objectives, and from that foundation, build the methods by which to measure progress toward and attainment of targeted outcomes. When setting those targets, it is helpful to consider the different levels of the outcomes, recognizing that the evaluation may not collect data at all levels.

One of the most popular evaluation models used for assessing the effectiveness of training and education programs is that of Kirkpatrick. The focus of this four-level model is to assess (1) reaction or satisfaction to the program, (2) learning from the program, (3) changes in learner behavior, and (4) program results or impact in its larger context.[12] Moore and colleagues expanded the Kirkpatrick framework from four to seven levels by incorporating elements specific to continuing medical education. This expanded framework includes adding participation as the lowest level of evaluation and building the highest levels with patient and community health as supplementary levels of impact.[13] The latter may be particularly helpful for educators when evaluating their students' value-added experiences.

The first level of the modified framework is participation, where we recognize that if learners do not show up and participate in the activity, they will likely have difficulty comprehending the material and may not learn at all. This is particularly true for some courses in the curriculum that do not require mandatory attendance. The second level of the schema is satisfaction. To assess learner reactions to the program, evaluators might ask students in a postsurvey what they thought about the program, what aspects were valuable, and what improvements might be needed. The third level of evaluation is learning. This level is both

TABLE 3.2   Modified Kirkpatrick and Moore Framework

Evaluation Framework	Description	Sources of Data
Participation level	Number of students who participated	Registration or attendance records
Satisfaction level	Degree to which the expectations of the participants were met	Subjective: Questionnaires completed by participants after activity
Learning level	Degree to which participants demonstrate knowing what or how the activity intended them to know	Objective: Pre- and posttests of knowledge Subjective: Self-report of knowledge gained
Performance level	Degree to which participants do what the activity intended them to be able to do	Objective: Observation of performance in patient care setting; scoring projects Subjective: Self-report of ability to perform or performance
Patient health level	Degree to which the health status of patients improves due to activities of participants	Objective: Health status measures recorded in patient charts or administrative databases Subjective: Patient self-report of health status
Community health level	Degree to which the health status of a community of patients changes due to changes in the practice behavior of participants	Objective: Epidemiological data and reports Subjective: Community self-report

Adapted from Moore DE, Green JS, Gallis HA. Achieving desired results and improved outcomes: Integrating planning and assessment throughout learning activities. *J Contin Educ Health Prof.* 2009;29:1–15. https://doi.org/10.1002/chp. PMID: 19288562. Note: These authors included level 4 of competence—"shows how"—which was excluded from this schema because that level is often assessed via simulation.

declarative in nature (knows) and procedural (knows how). Moore proposes that this level might be measured either subjectively by asking students if they learned or by asking evaluators to use an objective measure of learning through assessment (e.g., pre-/posttest of knowledge). The fourth level evaluates competence, where students demonstrate a skill or ability that the program intended for them to learn. Competence might be measured through objective observation of an activity or subjective self-reports. The fifth level of Moore's model includes changes in behavior or performance of students involved in the value-added activity in a real-life setting. Like other levels of the evaluation framework, this outcome can be measured objectively or subjectively via participant self-report surveys that ask whether the activity changed their behavior. Although subjective measures are appropriate, a more reliable outcome would involve direct measurement of performance through various assessment methods, such as direct observation, global assessments, checklists, and rubric scoring of projects.

Moore further builds on Kirkpatrick's model by including patient health and community health as supplementary levels of impact.[13] These additions convey that the activity is deemed effective if the outcomes include higher-level impacts that can be evaluated using patient-related measures, such as improved health. Similarly,

measuring the improved health of populations might include noting changes in epidemiology reports and/or related data that can be attributed in some way to the implementation of safety measures with a student value-added program. This approach of focusing on patients and community health is particularly helpful in evaluating value-added student programs since the goal is not just focused on student learning but also the impact upon the health system, patients, and the population. Table 3.2 summarizes the modified levels of Moore's framework as based on Kirkpatrick's model.[13]

The modified Kirkpatrick and Moore evaluation frameworks share some overlap with student assessment frameworks, which we will address next.

OVERALL OUTCOMES AND CONNECTIONS TO THE ASSESSMENT OF LEARNING

It is important to align assessments *for* learning (formative) and *of* learning (summative) with the objectives and program evaluation plan of the value-added program. **Assessment** is an iterative process, intended to provide useful feedback about what and how well students are learning. In this way, assessment data connect to the goals, objectives, and evaluation of the value-added program. Coordinating these efforts and using data for quality improvement (QI) cycles is an informative and effective approach.

Some educators use Miller's pyramid of clinical competency to focus learning and assessment at a specific scaffolded level.[14] A learner must first *know* what to do. This level includes the acquisition and interpretation of facts and information or declarative knowledge. The next level for Miller is *knows how*. Called **procedural knowledge**, it refers to when the learner describes how to do something but may not be able to actually do it. The third level is *shows how*; learners are expected to demonstrate how to do the task that they have learned. The final level according to Miller is *does*, which refers to learners using the knowledge and skills that they have developed in their practice and work. Examples of assessment types for each level are provided in Table 3.3.

Finally, a good illustration of the cycle of assessment (Fig. 3.3) and its relation to a program's overall goals or outcomes is provided by the Office of Academic Planning and Assessment at George Washington University.[15] A major strength of this particular assessment cycle is its consistency with Miller's pyramid, as both include (1) identifying what students should know and/or be able to do when they complete the program, (2) developing assessment strategies to measure the type and quality of learning expected, and (3) applying knowledge and demonstrating skills that are linked to the program goals or outcomes. Results of the assessments are incorporated back into the educational

cycle via an action plan aimed at improving learning and reducing knowledge gaps.

The intentional development of integrated formative and summative assessments, their importance, and relation to other program elements such as program evaluation are discussed throughout this field book. In Chapter 2, assessment is described as fostering engagement, involvement, and investment in an activity linked to learning, with key factors being relevance, authenticity, autonomy, collaboration, higher-order thinking skills, and self-assessment.

TABLE 3.3 Examples of Assessments Appropriate for Miller's Levels of Competence	
Level of Learning	**Types of Assessment**
Knows	Written examinations (multiple choice questions, true/false)
Knows how	Case presentation essays
Shows	Simulations, working through problems or cases, patient logs, objective structured clinical examination (OSCE)
Does	Direct observation workplace-based assessment, assessments of projects

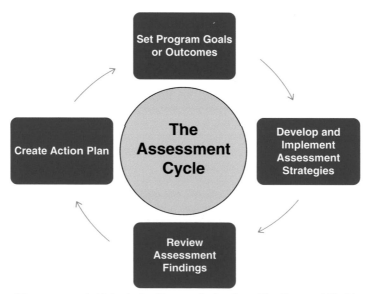

Fig. 3.3 Cycle of Assessment. (Adapted with permission from The George Washington University Office of Academic Planning and Assessment.)

Chapter 4 describes health systems science assessment development and the importance of connections to curricular development and value-added elements of learning opportunities. Chapter 6 describes a community program with a multimodal approach to student assessment, based on Miller. Finally, Chapter 8 describes how evaluation data revealed the misalignment of knowledge-based assessments. These examples of assessment approaches further illustrate the ways in which medical education programs utilize assessments that complement the institution's evaluation efforts.

ENGAGING STAKEHOLDERS IN PROGRAM EVALUATION

As noted throughout this chapter, when evaluating a value-added medical education program, we must remember to engage stakeholders throughout the process. In alignment with the utilization-focused evaluation approach, we consider internal and external stakeholders to be the intended users of evaluation findings; thus, we need to begin communications with those stakeholders at the program planning stage (well before activities are implemented). All too often, and to the detriment of the program, evaluation considerations and stakeholder opinions are sought after the program is already underway. "Whose opinion matters?" and "What would really be meaningful to them?" are two of the most important questions to ask in an evaluation.[16] Thus, evaluation questions (posed in a prior section of this chapter) and stakeholder input need to be considered at the onset of program planning.

When communicating with stakeholders at the program planning stage, leaders should ascertain the interests and needs of stakeholders that relate to the program's stated mission and goals. Regarding needs related to value-added medical education, program developers must first ensure that stakeholders understand the goals of the program and the outcomes of interest to the educational institution. This information will help stakeholders (1) understand how the program's anticipated outcomes align with the program goals, (2) align their own goals and reporting needs to those of the medical education program, and (3) realize the internal assumptions and program-specific contextual considerations that were made when developing the program. Understanding the latter will allow stakeholders to have more realistic expectations when it comes to evaluation findings.

Stakeholder input early in the program planning process can serve as an invaluable resource for institutions implementing value-added medical education activities. For example, preceptors at a teaching hospital may have acquired knowledge about innovative ways to engage students in value-added experiential activities based on their experiences with other medical schools, coupled with their understanding of the complex and ever-changing health care system. This insight may further inform the development of program activities that have the potential to affect goal-oriented impacts and outcomes; therefore, stakeholder input should be incorporated into the initial evaluation plan.

During the program implementation phase, stakeholders should receive timely updates about major programmatic changes and the potential impact of those changes. At the same time, program developers can inquire about any changes in stakeholder expectations and/or intended uses of evaluation findings. Engagement during the implementation phase can also provide stakeholders with additional opportunities to share new insights and provide ongoing assessment of the program's perceived value as a part of a formative evaluation process. Once evaluation findings are available, stakeholders should be provided with the results as outlined in the evaluation plan. Stakeholders can then use those findings for their own internal needs, while providing feedback about the utility of the information provided and changes that are recommended for program improvement.

CONCLUSIONS

Program evaluation is an essential component of value-added medical education. Medical educators need to take several steps in order to develop a comprehensive evaluation that demonstrates program success. First, educators and stakeholders need to consider a core set of questions that align with their value added educational goals, expected outcomes, and anticipated impacts. By asking these questions early in the process, educators will be equipped to devise an evaluation plan that incorporates the best approaches, methods, frameworks, and tools for a given program. Because of the dynamic nature of the evaluation process, the evaluation plan can be edited once the program has been implemented to reflect changes over time and to refocus on other outcomes and impacts. Using the findings from a robust evaluation, medical educators will be better prepared to identify areas of success, as well as those in need of improvement, and prioritize educational activities that highlight the value that medical students add to the health care team.

TAKE-HOME POINTS

1. Medical education evaluation is a systematic method of collecting and analyzing data to determine whether a program or activity is meeting its stated objectives.

2. Systematic, utilization-focused evaluation focuses on quality and effectiveness, incorporating measures that align with interests and expectations of internal and external stakeholders.

3. When developing an evaluation plan, asking "what," "how," and "why" questions is important. What is the activity or program to be evaluated, and how do identified outcomes link back to original objectives? How will the program be designed and implemented, and how does this impact my evaluation plan? Why is the program needed, and what gaps will it fill?

4. It is important to align evaluation methodologies and assessments *for* learning (formative) and *of* learning (summative) with objectives of value-added programs.

5. Implementing program improvements based on assessment data via quality improvement cycles coordinates and connects assessments with the objectives, outcomes, and program evaluation.

6. Stakeholders should have early input into the program planning process in order to leverage their expertise and set realistic expectations of evaluation results. During the implementation phase, timely updates to stakeholders will provide continuous improvement opportunities and maintain open communication.

QUESTIONS FOR FURTHER THOUGHT

1. How will the COVID-19 pandemic impact medical education evaluation in the long run?

2. How will medical education evaluation procedures evolve with advances in health care and technology?

3. What are some methods that we can use to evaluate student-led quality improvement initiatives? What value do medical students bring to a quality improvement committee?

4. What considerations need to be made when evaluating combined (dual) degree programs (e.g., MD/MPH, MD/MS) and physician scholar programs (i.e., MD/PhD, DO/PhD)? How do we determine the added value that these students bring to a health care team?

5. What are some unique challenges in developing medical education evaluation plans for colleges/schools with regional campuses?

6. How might assessment and evaluation data be used to improve medical education pedagogy while also solidifying the learners' understanding of their impact on patient and population health?

ANNOTATED BIBLIOGRAPHY

National Center for Chronic Disease Prevention and Health Promotion. *Developing an Effective Evaluation Plan: Setting the Course for Effective Program Evaluation.* Centers for Disease Control and Prevention. http://www.cdc.gov/obesity/downloads/CDC-Evaluation-Workbook-508.pdf. Published 2011. Accessed December 11, 2020.

This guidebook describes a six-step framework that can be used to guide evaluation planning efforts and the successful implementation of evaluation activities. The document outlines the core elements of an evaluation plan, logic model, and communication plan that can be used to disseminate findings and lessons learned.

World Health Organization. *WHO Evaluation Practice Handbook.* World Health Organization Publishing. https://apps.who.int/iris/handle/10665/96311. Published 2013. Accessed December 11, 2020.

This handbook provides step-by-step guidance for evaluation planning. The World Health Organization discusses the appropriate use of an evaluation process for quality improvement and identifies assessments that can be utilized along with other evaluation procedures.

Giancola SP. *Program Evaluation: Embedding Evaluation Into Program Design and Development.* Newbury Park, CA: SAGE Publications, Inc; 2020.

This book gives an overview of the evaluation process and provides practical guidance on how to conduct comprehensive evaluations for quality improvement purposes. The author also advises on how to use evaluation data to drive decision-making processes.

WK Kellogg Foundation. *Using Logic Models to Bring Together Planning, Evaluation, and Action: Logic Model Development Guide.* https://www.wkkf.org/resource-directory/resources/2004/01/logic-model-development-guide. Published January 2004. Accessed December 11, 2020.

This guidebook introduces the program logic model as a tool for evaluation planning and provides examples, checklists, and templates that can be used during the process. Guidance is also provided on how to expand basic logic models and apply modeling techniques that inform the selection elements to be included in an evaluation plan.

Moore DE, Green JS, Gallis HA. Achieving desired results and improved outcomes: Integrating planning and assessment throughout learning activities. *J Contin Educ Health Prof.* 2009;29:1–15. https://doi:10.1002/chp.20001. PMID: 19288562.

This article discusses various methods that can be used to plan and assess continuing medical education programs. The authors propose an expanded (seven-level) outcomes framework (based on the four-level Kirkpatrick model) that can be used for evaluation planning and implementation. Participation is added at the lowest level of evaluation, and patient and community health are included as supplementary levels.

REFERENCES

1. Association of American Medical Colleges and Liaison Committee on Medical Education. Functions and Structure of a Medical School: Standards for Accreditation of Medical Education Programs Leading to the MD

Degree. Washington, DC: LCME; 2020. https://lcme.org/publications/. Published March 2020. Accessed December 11.

2. Centers for Disease Control and Prevention. *Program Evaluation*. https://www.cdc.gov/eval/index.htm. Published May 20, 2019. Accessed December 11, 2020.

3. Vassar M, Wheeler DL, Davison M, Franklin J. Program evaluation in medical education: an overview of the utilization-focused approach. *J Educ Eval Health Prof*. 2010;7:1. https://doi.org/10.3352/jeehp.2010.7.1. PMID: 20559515.

4. Centers for Disease Control and Prevention Framework for program evaluation in public health. *MMWR*. 1999;48 (No. RR-11):4–31.

5. National Center for Chronic Disease Prevention and Health Promotion. *Developing an Effective Evaluation Plan: Setting the Course for Effective Program Evaluation*. Centers for Disease Control and Prevention; 2020. http://www.cdc.gov/obesity/downloads/CDC-Evaluation-Workbook-508.pdf. Published 2011. Accessed December 11.

6. World Health Organization. *WHO Evaluation Practice Handbook*. World Health Organization Publishing. https://apps.who.int/iris/handle/10665/96311. Published 2013. Accessed December 11, 2020.

7. Whelan AJ, Prescott J, Young G, Catanese VM, McKinney R. American Association of Medical Colleges. COVID-19: Guidance on Medical Students' Participation in Direct In-Person Patient Contact Activities. https://www.aamc.org/system/files/2020-08/meded-August-14-Guidance-on-Medical-Students-on-Clinical Rotations.pdf. Published August 14, 2020. Accessed December 11, 2020.

8. Mertens DM, ed. *Research and Evaluation in Education and Psychology: Integrating Diversity with Quantitative,*
Qualitative, and Mixed Methods. 5th ed. Los Angeles, CA: SAGE Publications, Inc; 2019.

9. Giancola SP. *Program Evaluation: Embedding Evaluation Into Program Design and Development*. Newbury Park, CA: SAGE Publications, Inc; 2020.

10. WK Kellogg Foundation. *Using Logic Models to Bring Together Planning, Evaluation, and Action: Logic Model Development Guide*. https://www.wkkf.org/resource-directory/resources/2004/01/logic-model-development-guide. Published January 2004. Accessed December 11, 2020.

11. Centers for Disease Control and Prevention, Program Performance and Evaluation Office. Program Evaluation Framework Checklist for Step 2. https://www.cdc.gov/eval/steps/step2/index.htm. Updated December 12, 2018. Accessed December 11, 2020.

12. Kirkpatrick D, Kirkpatrick J. *Evaluating Training Programs: The Four Levels*. San Francisco, CA: Berrett-Koehler Publishers; 1998.

13. Moore DE, Green JS, Gallis HA. Achieving desired results and improved outcomes: Integrating planning and assessment throughout learning activities. *J Contin Educ Health Prof*. 2009;29:1–15. https://doi.org/10.1002/chp.20001. PMID: 19288562.

14. Miller GE. The assessment of clinical skills/competence/performance. *Acad Med*. 1990;65(9 suppl):S63–S67. https://doi.org/10.1097/00001888-199009000-00045. PMID: 2400509.

15. The George Washington University, Office of Academic Planning and Assessment. *The Assessment Cycle*. https://assessment.gwu.edu/assessment-cycle. Published February 6, 2014. Accessed December 11, 2020.

16. Cook DA. Twelve tips for evaluating educational programs. *Med Teach*. 2010;32(4):296–301. https://doi.org/10.3109/01421590903480121. PMID: 20353325.

Practice/Preclerkship, Clerkship, and Longitudinal Experiences

Part II, *Practice*, highlights seven exemplar value-added medical education programs from around the United States. These programs are all administered by schools in the American Medical Association's Accelerating Change in Medical Education Consortium. The seven institutions represented have launched successful programs with a variety of local partners and a wide range of experiences for medical students. These experiences include students as patient navigators and care coordinators and as participants in clinical microsystems. Others involve students participating in community-based service-oriented education as health coaches and educators doing home visits or as embedded clinicians and advocates in community health centers throughout the country. Several programs utilize students as quality improvement champions and project leaders. All of the programs outlined have provided descriptions of their curricula, learning goals, assessment and evaluation strategies, resources needed, implementation histories, and key advice for feasibility and sustainability.

4

Students as Patient Navigators: The Penn State College of Medicine

Ami L. DeWaters, Barbara Blatt, Deanna Dubots, and Jed D. Gonzalo

LEARNING OBJECTIVES

1. Discuss how a patient navigation program can add value to individual patients, the health system, and to students' education.
2. Describe challenges that can arise in a patient navigation program.
3. Examine the importance of an interprofessional network in the development of a patient navigation program.

OUTLINE

CHAPTER SUMMARY

We describe the implementation of a patient navigation program for first-year medical students at Penn State College of Medicine. The program is a part of the health systems science curriculum for the medical school and provides the experiential component for learning key concepts, such as social determinants of health, health care policy, health care structures and processes, and health care improvement. The program utilizes resources from both the medical school and the health system and relies on expertise from an interdisciplinary cohort of mentors and faculty. This chapter outlines benefits from and challenges to the implementation of such a program in the undergraduate medical education setting.

INTRODUCTION

From the inception of the **patient navigation** program at Penn State College of Medicine (PSCOM), we aimed to ensure that participating medical students would add value to the health care system as well as have value added to their own education. In fact, we designed the patient navigation program specifically with those goals in mind. The program began as a component of a larger curriculum that was written for the American Medical Association (AMA) Accelerating Change in Medical Education grant. That grant established **health systems science** (HSS) as the fourth pillar of medical education at PSCOM, complementing the basic and clinical sciences and health humanities.

The 18-month longitudinal HSS curriculum is offered in the first 2 years of medical school at PSCOM. The curriculum focuses on developing knowledge, skills, and attitudes in 12 key domains (see Fig. 1.4), including population health management, health policy, health information technology, high-value care, health care structures and process, and health systems improvement. This didactic course exists in the formal classroom setting. However, to provide students with the opportunity to experientially learn the concepts discussed in the classroom, we integrated the formal coursework with an experiential student patient navigator component. This role immersed students in the clinical environment immediately and gave them the opportunity to learn from patients and interprofessional clinicians about the health care delivery system and HSS concepts.

Patient navigation is a relatively new concept in medicine. It began in response to the findings from the 1989 American Cancer Society National Hearings on Cancer in the Poor, which outlined the significant challenges patients in poverty faced when attempting to seek care for cancer.[1] Dr. Harold Freeman launched the first patient navigation program in 1990 in Harlem, New York, in an attempt to address these challenges. Implementation of this program dramatically improved health outcomes in a population of patients with breast cancer at Harlem Hospital Center. After proven success, patient navigation programs began to emerge across the United States. Performed by an individual with a distinct role on a health care team, the key principles of patient navigation include:

1. focusing care on patients and their needs;
2. integrating access to resources to meet the needs of patients interacting with a fragmented system;
3. seeking to eliminate or prevent barriers;
4. facilitating care across sites and locations; and
5. coordinating care.[1]

These principles align with many of the principles of HSS. In the coursework, students are asked to think broadly about how barriers to care—for example, health care disparities or financial challenges—may affect a patient's health. In the context of a patient navigation program, the students are able to help actual patients overcome those exact barriers. This experience not only helps facilitate the students' learning of these principles, but patients in need also receive assistance.

DESCRIPTION OF PATIENT NAVIGATION AT PENN STATE COLLEGE OF MEDICINE

The patient navigation program was launched at PSCOM in 2014. Each first-year medical student is assigned a patient navigator mentor, who works at a designated clinical site with identified site-specific needs for navigation. The student receives training in navigation during the first month of the HSS curriculum. The training includes social history taking, communication training with a standardized patient, identifying and understanding **social determinants of health**, poverty simulation, and a beginning exposure to the expectation of a physician's role and to the core principles of professionalism. After a month of in-classroom education, students begin work at their clinical sites and meet the assigned mentor for a site-specific orientation. PSCOM had 18 different clinical sites for the academic year 2020 to 2021. These sites include skilled nursing facilities, acute and subacute rehabilitation facilities, primary care clinics, and subspecialty clinics (Table 4.1). The mentor for each site describes the patient navigation program to the assigned students. The mentor also describes how the program has been specifically developed in collaboration with the HSS team, the clinical site, and the care team for that site.

Additionally, during orientation, the site mentor reviews community resources that may be helpful for students when they are working directly with their patients in need. The mentor assigns each student a patient or patients who would benefit from navigation. Initially, a single patient is assigned to two students to incorporate a collaborative learning component and as an additional safety measure (e.g., during home visits). The goal is for students to be able to develop longitudinal and meaningful relationships with several patients over the course of the year. In addition to being able to solicit patients' underlying barriers to care through home visits, telephone calls, and asynchronous communication, students utilize the site mentor and electronic health record (EHR) in assessing their assigned patients' health care barriers. Students spend approximately 8 to 12 hours each month participating in the patient navigation program.

With guidance from the site mentor, student patient navigators perform tasks in three main categories:

1. Providing information and education for patients and their families (e.g., social care plan and available community resources);
2. Offering emotional and psychological support; and
3. Facilitating coordination and continuity of care for their patients.

In the first 6 years of the program, approximately 800 medical students have provided patient navigation services for approximately 5000 patients in the 5-county area surrounding PSCOM in southcentral Pennsylvania. While explicit health outcomes for these patients are anecdotal (and under investigation), we have been able to identify the structural and social determinants of health

TABLE 4.1   Description of Clinical Sites Utilized in Patient Navigation Program

Site Name	Number of Students	Type of Setting	Profession of Mentor(s)
Penn State Health Primary Care Clinics*	30	University	Social Worker
Penn State Health Acute Rehabilitation Facility*	28	University	Clinical Case Manager
Post-Acute Care Skilled Nursing Facilities*	24	Community	Advanced Practice Providers and Physician
Beacon Clinic (Primary Care)	2	Community	Nurse Care Coordinator and Social Worker
Geisinger Holy Spirit Inpatient Hospital	6	Community	Nurse Care Coordinator
Lebanon VA Inpatient Hospital	4	University	Physician
Lebanon Valley Free Clinic (Primary Care)	2	Community	Nurse Care Coordinator
Pennsylvania Psychiatric Institute (Inpatient)	4	University	Nurse Care Coordinator
Penn State Health Breast Clinic	4	University	Physician
Penn State Health Community Paramedics	8	University	Paramedic
Penn State Health Eating Disorders Clinic	2	University	Social Worker and Physician
Penn State Health Internal Medicine Clinic (Primary Care)	4	University	Physician
Penn State Health Pediatrics Clinic (Primary Care)	4	University	Nurse Care Coordinator
Penn State Health SCOPE (gastrointestinal subspecialty clinic)	4	University	Physician
YMCA–Harrisburg	2	Community	Case Worker
WellSpan Sechler Cancer Center	2	Community	Nurse Care Coordinator and Social Worker
Penn State Health Preanesthesia Clinic	2	University	Social Worker
Penn State Health Medical Group (Primary Care)	2	University	Physician

*Hub sites, implemented in 2016 to help build sustainability for the program.

that are prevalent in our five-county catchment area. Throughout the year, students submit written logs for their patient encounters and delineate in those logs which structural and social determinants of health are present for their patient. Social isolation, transportation issues, and lack of access to mental health services are the most prevalent structural and social determinants of health. All play a significant role in generating barriers to health care. This information has been considered valuable to Penn State Health in discussions focused on improving care delivery and meeting the needs of patients in different regions and demographic groups. As a result, the patient navigation program has been able to demonstrate its value not only to the individual patient who receives assistance, but also to the system as it strives to engage in population health management.[2]

For students, this program is the primary early clinical experience—their first introduction to the clinical setting. Therefore, it is their first integration into the medical profession. The program helps to facilitate their professional identity formation early in their undergraduate medical education.[3] Complementing the other areas of the curriculum—including the health humanities—PSCOM students have identified this program as an opportunity to participate in and learn how to engage in improvement of care delivery and caring for patients holistically.[3]

LEARNING GOALS OF THE PROGRAM

The learning goals for the patient navigation program purposely span the Accreditation Council for Graduate Medical Education six core competencies: patient care, medical knowledge, professionalism, systems-based practice, interpersonal communication skills, and practice-based learning and improvement (Table 4.2). We believe that only through early immersion in the clinical learning environment can students truly begin to develop knowledge,

TABLE 4.2   Patient Navigation Entrustable Professional Activities (EPA) Mapped to Core Competencies

	Systems-Based Practice	Interpersonal Communication and Skills	Patient Care	Medical Knowledge	Practice-Based Learning and Improvement	Professionalism
EPA 1: Interact professionally with patients, staff, and clinicians in both informal and clinically based settings.					X	
EPA 2: Effectively manage communication with patients and members of the interprofessional care team.		X				
EPA 3: Comprehensively assess and diagnose the root causes of a patient's health care situation.	X		X	X		
EPA 4: Identify and facilitate linkage of health system and community resources for patients in need.	X		X			
EPA 5: Participate in and contribute to the ongoing work of an interprofessional care team within a clinical setting.		X	X		X	X
EPA 6: Document patient encounters in the electronic health record in a timely and accurate manner.		X				X
EPA 7: Apply the habits of a system thinker when they work to address patients' health care situation.	X		X		X	
EPA 8: Build a therapeutic relationship with a patient.		X	X			X

skills, and attitudes in each of these domains. Therefore, the patient navigation program uniquely adds value to first-year students' education because it allows them to gain aptitude in these domains in a way that standard, didactic coursework in the early years of undergraduate medical education does not.[4] Additionally, this learning helps improve the transition into the clerkship and post-clerkship phases of the students' learning.

The overarching learning goal is for students to demonstrate a holistic approach to health care, including biopsychosocial and systems-based elements, while participating as proactive change agents in the health care delivery system. By the end of the program, students are entrusted to:

1. Interact professionally with patients, staff, and clinicians in both informal and clinically based settings.
2. Effectively manage communication with patients and members of the interprofessional care team.
3. Comprehensively assess and diagnose the root causes of a patient's health care situation.
4. Identify and facilitate linkage of health system and community resources for patients in need.
5. Participate in and contribute to the ongoing work of an interprofessional care team within a clinical setting.
6. Document patient encounters in the EHR in a timely and accurate manner.
7. Apply the habits of a **systems thinker** when they work to address patients' health care situations.
8. Build a therapeutic relationship with a patient.

ASSESSMENT TECHNIQUES FOR MEDICAL STUDENTS PARTICIPATING AS NAVIGATORS

The expansive set of learning goals and entrustable professional activities outlined earlier necessitate multimodal assessment tools for the students. First, as with many clinically based experiences, the student's professional site mentor completes an assessment of each student's performance. There is one assessment at the mid-year, which is formative. The final assessment occurs at the end of the year, which is summative. Site mentor evaluations are used to particularly evaluate communication skills, professional attributes, teamwork, collaboration, and ability to build relationships with patients.

Second, there are several small groups in the HSS coursework dedicated to debriefing students' patient navigation experiences. In these sessions, students are asked to use their experiences to reflect and discuss the following: their roles at the patient navigation site; observations of patients, clinicians, and staff at the site; the habits of a systems thinker they used or observed during their experiences;

and any ethnographic observations of their health systems experiences, elicited by prompts. Ethnographic prompts included in this activity relate to social determinants of health, population health, policy, public health, and value-based care. These activities are evaluated by their small-group facilitators, who are different faculty from their site mentors. These small-group facilitators are in a position to more explicitly assess students' system thinking skills within the classroom and in the reflections on their patient navigator experiences.

Finally, throughout the program, students are asked to complete narrative logs of experiences with individual patients with whom they have worked during navigation. These logs ask for students to identify and discuss the patient's structural and social determinants of health, the health care team's and their personal challenges to providing care for this patient, and the system thinking skills the student has learned and applied to assist the patient. These logs are reviewed by the course directors and allow students to be assessed for their ability to comprehensively assess a patient's health care situation.

This combination of assessment tools has been extraordinarily meaningful, both for students and PSCOM. These assessment tools have become a key means of quickly identifying students who may be struggling with professionalism expectations or communication skills, which may predict future performance in clinical clerkships. Through early identification of struggling learners, students are able to have performance improvement plans developed promptly and thereby prevent struggles from occurring later in their medical education. PSCOM now relies on these assessment tools, particularly for the domains of professionalism and communication.

PROCEDURES FOR EVALUATION OF THE NAVIGATION PROGRAM

The patient navigation program is rigorously evaluated annually. Data collected through program evaluation activities serve dual purposes. First, these data enable us to examine curriculum delivery in order to maintain quality standards and ensure compliance with accreditation requirements. Second, these data enable us to further our understanding of the effectiveness of the teaching methods. Due to the diversity of sites, patient populations, and mentors involved in the program, it is critical to ensure that each site receives individualized evaluation.

To that end, at the same time students receive evaluations from their site mentors (mid-year and end of year), they perform evaluations of their patient navigation site. These evaluations are reviewed carefully by the course directors and, if necessary, adjustments to site practices may be made mid-year. In addition, course directors meet with student curriculum representatives three times a year to ensure that any global concerns or feedback can be addressed. It is equally as critical to ensure that site mentors are given time and space to give feedback on the program. An annual retreat is held with all site mentors, who are specifically asked to comment on any areas in need of improvement and ways to enhance students' ability to add value to the mentors' sites.

From a more macrosystem perspective, patient navigation is also evaluated in its ability to contribute to meeting accreditation standards for PSCOM. Several accreditation items outlined by the Liaison Committee on Medical Education (LCME) are met largely by our program and are listed here.[5]

1. Service learning: Defined as "the faculty of a medical school ensure that the medical education program provides sufficient opportunities for, encourages, and supports medical student participation in service-learning and community service activities."

2. Societal principles: Defined as "the faculty of a medical school ensure that the medical curriculum includes instruction in the diagnosis, prevention, appropriate reporting, and treatment of the medical consequences of common societal problems."

3. Medical ethics: Defined as "describe the methods used to assess medical students' ethical behavior in the care of patients and to identify and remediate medical students' breaches of ethics in patient care."

4. Communication skills: Defined as "describe the specific educational activities, including student assessment, and the relevant learning objectives included in the curriculum."

5. Interpersonal collaborative skills: Defined as "the faculty of a medical school ensure that the core curriculum of the medical education program prepares medical students to function collaboratively on health care teams that include health professionals from other disciplines as they provide coordinated services to patients. These curricular experiences include practitioners and/or students from the other health professions. Provide three examples of required experiences where medical students are brought together with students or practitioners from other health professions to learn to function collaboratively on health care teams with the goal of providing coordinated services to patients."[5]

The program is evaluated annually to ensure that it continues to satisfy these standards. The ability of the program to help meet LCME requirements has added to its value for PSCOM.

NECESSARY RESOURCES TO BUILD A PATIENT NAVIGATION PROGRAM

Those considering implementing a patient navigation program need to be aware that it is resource intensive. We found it imperative to have a dedicated program coordinator, ideally someone who has a Master of Education degree (or health administration, etc.). The coordinator oversees all site mentors and collaborates with them to develop site-specific navigation programs, ensuring that each mentor is clear on the expectations and goals of the program. The coordinator also provides support to the mentors, identifies program best practices, problem solves with the site as issues arise, designs and implements changes within each site, and is available to answer questions and provide educational guidance. It is important for the patient navigation coordinator to participate in site visits in order to better understand how that clinical unit operates within the health system and effectively identify the program needs. All administrative responsibilities, such as obtaining the necessary background clearances and vaccination records for the students, are handled by the program coordinator in collaboration with the Office of Student Affairs. For us, the coordinator has also been critical in linking the HSS curriculum into the patient navigation curriculum so that experiential learning of classroom material can occur.

In addition to the coordinator, faculty who are willing and able to serve as site mentors are necessary (Fig. 4.1). For the patient navigation network, we have been privileged to work with engaged and action-oriented clinical site mentors and champions. Without these individuals, the idea of patient navigation would have never become reality. These faculty include nursing care coordinators, social workers, physicians, and care managers. The mentors identify patients in need of navigation and guide students on how to integrate into the interprofessional clinical team. While some faculty may be able to mentor a small number of students on a volunteer basis, many faculty who mentor 20 or more students require some form of salary support to participate. The number of mentors required depends on class size and the number of students each mentor can accommodate. The number of clinical sites necessary varies between different medical schools based on class size and number of mentors available. Therefore, there must be enough clinical sites, each with a patient population willing to engage in patient navigation, within a reasonable driving distance of the school.

These interdisciplinary mentors and the interdisciplinary staff who participate in the program at each clinical site have been a great addition to the education of the medical

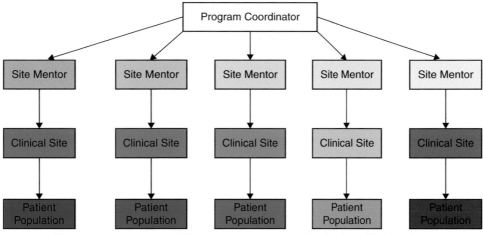

Fig. 4.1 Framework of Necessary Resources for Patient Navigation.

students. We have found that students rate their nonphysician mentors more highly than physician mentors in communication frequency, importance to work, and education. Students also report that nonphysician mentors are more likely to focus on HSS concepts when teaching, such as social determinants of health and challenges in health care delivery.[6] The navigation program provides a venue to allow students to learn from these interdisciplinary mentors in a way that is not possible elsewhere in their medical education.

Along with health care professionals, the patient navigation program requires investment from the community. Students need to be aware of the resources that exist in order to effectively help patients address any barriers they may encounter. PSCOM community partners have been invaluable in engaging in the patient navigation program and educating the students on the many programs they provide, from food pantries to transportation services to in-home medical services.

Patient navigation also requires the resource investment of time. In order for students to meaningfully assist patients in the clinical setting, they must commit a reasonable amount of time to patient navigation weekly. As mentioned earlier in this chapter, students work a couple of hours a week, with a requirement to invest 8 to 12 hours a month in the program. Since the program operates September through May, there is approximately a 100-hour time commitment for the year. In a medical school curriculum that has multiple competing priorities, it is essential that the program be given the space it needs in the curriculum to allow students to participate without too much additional stress.

THE IMPLEMENTATION HISTORY AND STRATEGIES EMPLOYED

When patient navigation was first implemented in 2014, it was based strongly on the foundation of the HSS curriculum. That curriculum and its 12 competency domains served as the theoretical framework in which navigation was grounded. If in the classroom we were discussing insurance and underinsured and uninsured populations, then, in navigation, students were supposed to be assisting patients who were underinsured or uninsured as they sought medical care. As the program has grown over the last 6 years, we learned to make the links between the classroom and navigation as the experiential component as explicit as possible. To accomplish that link, classes now frequently start with students sharing experiences from navigation. In addition, the documentation and logs that students submit ask them to specifically outline how they applied what they learned in class to their patients assigned in navigation. So-called "huddles" have also been implemented at navigation sites. Mentors meet with their students as a group to discuss challenges they are having while navigating for their patients, and the mentors take the opportunity to highlight teaching points from class that week. We found that without these direct connections, students failed to relate the two components of the curriculum to one another.

While the theoretical framework used for navigation has not changed over the first 6-year period, our patient navigation has shifted from a program that was voluntary for students and involved over 40 sites to one that is mandatory and involves approximately 20 sites. The intention was always for the program to become mandatory. However, the speed with which the program had to be developed in the first year did not make it possible to secure enough sites and mentors for all students to participate. Therefore, it was necessary for the program to be limited to volunteers for the first year; about half of the class volunteered for the over 40 sites available for patient navigation. Since 2015, the patient navigation program has been mandatory for all first-year medical students.

Selection of sites was based on a number of factors. First, the site had to have an individual employed who was willing to serve as a dedicated mentor, usually without funding for the effort. Second, the site had to serve patients who required navigation. Third, the site had to be able to demonstrate that there would be navigation work available for students for the entire year. Site locations have shifted over the years; mentors may leave the site, navigation work may cease at the site, or the site may lose bandwidth to invest in navigation.

We continue to have challenges maintaining enough sites and mentors for all students. In 2016, in response to not having enough clinical sites, we developed an ethnographic program as an additional educational opportunity that we implemented for 4 months that year. As ethnographers, students participated in novel "ethnography" roles to observe and learn about the patient's experience of care within the system and were exposed to patient experiences in various health settings. Each ethnography student spent a maximum of 12 hours over a period of 3 weeks at each ethnography site. Ethnography sites were composed of the Penn State Hershey Emergency Department and various community-based sites, including the Salvation Army Rehabilitation Center, Christ Lutheran Church, Hope Lodge Hershey, and the Ronald McDonald Family Room. Students were taught the core ethnography skills to perform these roles prior to beginning them.

Starting in the spring of 2016, we developed a patient navigation mentor/clinical care manager role. This new role provided a solution to our barrier of not having enough patient navigation sites and mentors for all medical students. It was also the beginning of the shift in the program to the "hub" model (Fig. 4.2). With funding from the Penn State Hershey Health System and PSCOM, we created a patient navigation hub model to provide partial salary support for hub site mentors. The goals of the model included:

1. improving sustainability of the program;
2. partnering with individuals who provide exceptional education to the students and who have the capacity to mentor at least 20 students;
3. decreasing the variability at the sites; and
4. increasing communication between the school and program.

The hub model has been received very positively by students and mentors. It has increased consistency of experience

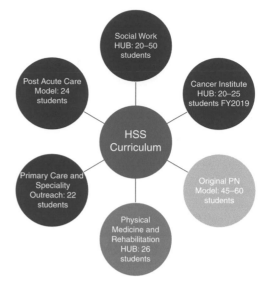

Fig. 4.2 The "Hub" Model for Patient Navigation. *HSS*, Health systems science.

between clinical sites, which we have found to be key in student satisfaction. Supporting mentors so that they may participate in multiple, consecutive years has also allowed for improvement in processes in the program. Therefore, the depth of involvement at each site has grown over time, and students are able to add more value than at the inception of the program.

The hub model would not have been possible without funding from PSCOM. In the beginning, our patient navigation program had only one funded role—the patient navigation coordinator. This role was initially funded in part by the aforementioned AMA grant. As the program demonstrated its value, PSCOM leadership decided to fund that role directly, as well as the patient navigation mentor/clinical care manager roles mentioned earlier.

KEY ADVICE FOR FEASIBILITY AND SUSTAINABILITY

One of the main challenges for us has been the ability to maintain enough clinical sites and mentors for the program. Through surveys and interviews with current and past site mentors, we have learned the main barriers and challenges to sustaining patient navigation sites.[7] These include structural changes within the clinic and health system (e.g., implementation of a new EHR) that made integration of students more challenging, an overestimation of the number of students a site could optimally mentor, mentor availability (e.g., mentor receives new role, changes employers), and interactions with less than engaged students leading to mentor burnout.

To overcome these barriers and challenges, it is essential to maintain consistent communication between the program coordinator and the site mentors. Developing a proactive, continuous quality improvement process between the program coordinator, course directors, students, and mentors is a necessity. Offering an annual retreat for site mentor collaboration is another way to help receive feedback, set expectations, and improve collaboration. The mentors and sites increasingly recognized the need for ongoing communication, collaboration, and sharing of ideas related to best practices to ensure that optimal conditions were created for learning and patient care. These regular check-ins, quality improvement processes, and retreats have been described as vital to making improvements and are also important for building a network and community between mentors.

The second main challenge encountered was a lack of depth and breadth of HSS teaching faculty who felt comfortable serving as mentors in the program. To address and potentially overcome this gap, we partnered with administrators of our health system to design, develop, and implement a health system-based faculty development program, the Health Systems Science Academy (HSSA). HSSA is an application-based faculty development program that provides participants with experiential learning opportunities in an environment that fosters intraprofessional team skills, curiosity, systems thinking, and a commitment to enhancing education and improving our systems of care. The systems-based curriculum integrates knowledge in six of the domains of health systems science, including (1) population and public health; (2) health care policy, economics, and management; (3) clinical informatics and health information technology; (4) value-based care; (5) health system improvement; and (6) health care delivery, structures, and processes. This program has helped ensure a consistent mental model among site mentors about the educational goals of the patient navigation program.

Finally, one of the most vital elements to achieve sustainability is to attain system-wide and community support and funding for the program. Key administrators in the implementation and success of our project include the dean of PSCOM, the corporate executive officer of Penn State Health, the vice dean for educational affairs, the chief financial officer, the vice president and chief quality officer, the vice president of operational excellence, the vice president of population health, the director of ambulatory nursing, the chief information officer, and many others. We leveraged key administrators by including them in the design, development, and implementation of the HSS curriculum, including the patient navigation program. System-wide education on the implementation of the new HSS programs is important for continuous integration and permeation throughout the entire health system. Partnership and collaboration with external health systems, community-based organizations, and other Pennsylvania health affiliations has also been an important facilitator to the success of our project. Multiple external health systems and community partners have been key in the success and sustainability of HSS education, especially the patient navigation component.

CONCLUSION

Patient navigation is a resource-intensive program that requires significant support from a multitude of partners in order to be successful. However, it is well worth the investment given the potential for benefits. From individual patients with additional resources to improve their health, to students with systems-minded identities and skills, to a health system with more information to guide population health management, patient navigation has the ability to add value in a myriad of ways.

STUDENT REFLECTIONS

As a student, one lacks an intimate understanding of the health care system. A student is in a unique position to both work for and learn from patients, in that the student also gains working knowledge of how the logistical side of the health care system operates. The patient navigation program puts the student in a position to experience the "dotting of i's and crossing of t's" in a patient's care that aren't addressed by the rest of the team. What results is the realization that there is a surprisingly wide range of tasks and barriers met by the patient themselves; this can be overwhelmingly difficult for patients who are already struggling with debilitating health conditions. Students become familiar with how to assist their patients to best meet their financial, emotional, and medical needs, and gain insight into the general obstacles faced by anyone seeking help from the health care system. We also offer a service to the patient by providing assistance in tasks such as arranging transportation for follow-up care, working with insurance companies for compensation, arranging for obtaining durable medical goods, and simply helping patients to understand what exactly is happening to them. The benefits therefore are twofold.

As a patient navigator, I was able to deeply involve myself with a level of patient care I simply wouldn't have the time to participate in as a resident or attending physician. From the confusing and heartbreaking early moments in processing a devastating diagnosis to the financial and personal struggles of arranging long-term care, the assistance a student can offer through patient navigation is a unique tool that is instrumental to learners and patients alike.

—Dennis Madden

REFERENCES

1. Freeman HP, Rodriguez RL. History and principles of patient navigation. *Cancer*. 2011;117(S15):3537–3540.
2. Gonzalo JD, Lucey C, Wolpaw T, Chang A. Value-added clinical systems learning roles for medical students that transform education and health: a guide for building partnerships between medical schools and health systems. *Acad Med*. 2017;92(5):602–607.
3. McDermott C, Shank K, Shervinskie C, Gonzalo JD. Developing a professional identity as a change agent early in medical school: the students' voice. *J Gen Intern Med*. 2019;34(5):750–753.
4. Gonzalo JD, Dekhtyar M, Hawkins RE, Wolpaw DR. How can medical students add value? Identifying roles, barriers, and strategies to advance the value of undergraduate medical education to patient care and the health system. *Acad Med*. 2017;92(9):1294–1301.
5. Liaison Committee on Medical Education. *Functions and Structure of Medical School*. Washington, DC: Liaison Committee on Medical Education; 2018. http://www.lcme.org/wp-content/uploads/filebase/articles/October-2017-The-75-Year-History-of-the-LCME_COLOR.pdf. Published March 2018. Accessed 18.12.20.
6. Gonzalo JD, Wolpaw D, Graaf D, Thompson BM. Educating patient-centered, systems-aware physicians: a qualitative analysis of medical student perceptions of value-added clinical systems learning roles. *BMC Med Educ*. 2018;18(1):248.
7. Gonzalo JD, Graaf D, Ahluwalia A, Wolpaw DR, Thompson BM. A practical guide for implementing and maintaining value-added clinical systems learning roles for medical students using a diffusion of innovations framework. *Adv Health Sci Educ Theory Pract*. 2018;23(4):699–720.

5

Students as Patient Navigators: Case Western Reserve University School of Medicine

Heidi L. Gullett

LEARNING OBJECTIVES

1. Describe a pragmatic example of a longitudinal community-based preclinical medical student health system navigation program.
2. Discuss key elements of context and program implementation facilitating value-added role(s) for students.
3. Identify opportunities at the interface of value-added roles and health systems science.
4. Highlight a timely example of value-added roles in the era of COVID-19 resulting from prior infrastructure and community relationships.

OUTLINE

CHAPTER SUMMARY

This chapter describes key elements of the Case Western Reserve University School of Medicine patient health system navigation program that began in 2016. Preclinical medical students who are matched with veterans at the Cleveland Veterans Affairs or newly arrived refugee families at Neighborhood Family Practice—a federally qualified community health center—partner with patients for a year, helping them navigate the health care system and address social service needs. The health system navigation program follows the foundational health systems science course entitled "Block 1: Becoming A Doctor," which occurs in the first month of medical school. In each of the two clinical settings, student patient navigators join the patient-centered medical home interprofessional care team, providing value-added roles across a variety of health systems science domains. This chapter also explores key contextual elements of the program that foster implementation and sustainability. Additionally, this chapter describes a novel example of value-added medical student roles in the Cuyahoga County COVID-19 response that resulted from the existing infrastructure and community relationships in the patient navigator program. Finally, the chapter includes considerations around resources, challenges, and future directions for research and program evaluation.

INTRODUCTION

Health professions students long for educational opportunities where their work provides value to the patients with whom they interact, the health systems where they learn, and the communities through which they rotate.[1] In traditional medical education models, students tend to function in apprentice or limited clinical roles alongside more seasoned clinicians rather than in a capacity that provides added value. Health professions students, however, possess tremendous potential to transform the systems in which they are placed while working toward competencies in numerous curricular domains.

The evolution of **health systems science** (HSS) as a foundational pillar of medical education creates an opportunity to rethink experiences for learners and challenges medical educators to design new models of care delivery inclusive of students in **value-added roles**.[2]

This chapter describes key elements of the Case Western Reserve University School of Medicine (CWRU SOM) patient health system navigation (PN) program that began in 2016. This chapter describes the program, explores key contextual elements that fostered implementation and highlights considerations around resources, student assessment, program evaluation, and sustainability. Several program vignettes are also included to illustrate impact.

DESCRIPTION OF PATIENT NAVIGATION AT CASE WESTERN RESERVE UNIVERSITY SCHOOL OF MEDICINE

The **patient navigator** program functions as a first-year elective in which preclinical medical students are matched with veterans at the Louis Stokes Cleveland Veterans Affairs (VA) Medical Center or with newly arrived refugee families at Neighborhood Family Practice (NFP), a **federally qualified community health center** (FQHC) in Cleveland, Ohio. Students are partnered with their patients for a year, helping them navigate the health care system and address social service needs. Students work longitudinally alone or in pairs.[3,4] They accompany patients to primary and specialty care appointments; coordinate with case managers, social service providers, pharmacies, and other community-based organizations; and help patients navigate an often complex and unforgiving health care system. Students who partner with patients at the Cleveland VA work within interprofessional patient-aligned care teams. Students at NFP join an interprofessional care team within the FQHC that, like the VA, is also designated as a patient-centered medical home. NFP provides a wide range of services, including refugee health screenings through the federal refugee resettlement program as well as primary care, maternity, behavioral health, dental, and pharmacy services to over 21,000 patients of all ages annually.

Students are required to interact with their partner patient or family through phone calls and home or office visits at a minimum once a month, but most participate more frequently to address needs. Students track their patient contacts and lessons learned via monthly logs. Students from both sites also meet with elective faculty monthly in supplemental learning sessions, where they share experiences and insights from their navigation roles and explore HSS content in more depth, building on their first block of medical school, which serves as the foundational HSS course known as Block 1.

Learning Goals of the Program

Learning goals for the patient navigator program include:
- To deepen understanding of multiple HSS content areas through community patient navigation experiences and monthly workshops.
- To engage in systems thinking and systems analysis to identify advocacy opportunities for different levels of patient and health care team needs.
- To identify health care needs of patients, develop coordination of care plans, and implement the plans using quality improvement methods.
- To integrate medical students into interprofessional teams so that they obtain pragmatic skills necessary for clinical systems navigation, including electronic health record (EHR) and interpreter training.
- To inspire reflection on the role of medical students and physicians in health systems change to positively impact individual and community health outcomes.

TECHNIQUES TO ASSESS LEARNERS

The HSS design team created the student assessments for all preclinical longitudinal community electives, including patient navigator, given that they all address HSS domains. As such, the HSS design team based the assessment on core competencies of the Interprofessional Education Collaborative (IPEC), which reflects that interprofessional education is a foundational domain of HSS.[5,6] The supervising faculty member completes assessments through direct observation, team feedback, and review of monthly student logs that document the frequency and type of contact, conditions addressed, and activities completed.

The assessment domains include[6]:
- Humanism: Place interests of patients and populations at the center of interprofessional health care delivery and population health programs and policies, with the goal of promoting health and health equity across the life span. (IPEC Values/Ethics Subcompetency)
- Longitudinal relationships: Develop a trusting relationship with patients, families, and other team members. (IPEC Values/Ethics Subcompetency)

- Professional engagement: Forge interdependent relationships with other professions within and outside of the health system to improve care and advance learning. (IPEC Roles/Responsibilities Subcompetency)
- Systems thinking: Engage health and other professionals in shared patient-centered and population-focused problem-solving. (IPEC Team and Teamwork Subcompetency)
- Teamwork: Work in cooperation with those who receive care, those who provide care, and others who contribute to or support the delivery of prevention and health services and programs. (IPEC Values/Ethics Subcompetency)
- Interprofessional Communication: Engage diverse professionals who complement one's own professional expertise, as well as associated resources, to develop strategies to meet specific health and health care needs of patients and populations. (IPEC Communication Subcompetency)

Students also complete the Systems Thinking Scale (STS) at the beginning and conclusion of the elective.[7] Given that students self-select for this elective, we have observed a ceiling effect in these scores as participating students tend to enter with a strong systems thinking approach following Block 1 and prior to starting the elective.

EVALUATION PROCEDURES

The primary source of program evaluation data thus far has been generated through focus groups with each student cohort conducted by a PhD qualitative research associate. The core HSS domains serve as the framework for a qualitative thematic analysis of these focus groups, along with quality improvement feedback to improve program logistics and efficiency.[2,5]

Future program evaluation will include assessment of the navigator impact on the clinical system and health care team, patient clinical and experience outcomes, and impact on student HSS subject exam performance, professional identity formation, and career specialty choice. Additionally, to scale and sustain the patient navigator program, further research and rigorous program evaluation is necessary on patient perception, community partner impact, cost-effectiveness, patient outcomes, model scalability, development and maintenance of effective community partnerships, and impact on systems thinking and professional identity formation.

RESOURCES NEEDED

The CWRU patient navigator program provides an important longitudinal HSS elective opportunity for early medical students, with demonstrated value for patients, health care teams, and health systems. However, this robust program requires immense faculty and staff support, as well as organizational commitment by both the SOM and community partners.

We successfully deployed this program because we had multiple levels of support, including from the AMA Accelerating Change in Medical Education Consortium. The consortium served as the catalyst for the initiation of this program, which was enhanced by partnership with Penn State College of Medicine and other schools that provided technical expertise and support for innovations in HSS. The program was also feasible due to a strong commitment from the CWRU SOM dean, who championed improvement in community health and innovations in medical education as two of the three SOM strategic priorities. As part of these strategic initiatives, the dean created two innovative faculty positions (assistant dean for health systems science and population health liaison with the Cuyahoga County Board of Health) within the SOM, which positioned the two faculty leads for this program to develop strategic partnerships with community organizations that agreed to devote resources to hosting students for the longitudinal navigator experience.

At a more granular level, our program is also made possible by a dedicated administrator who works closely with the assistant dean for HSS, functions as a course manager for Block 1, and coordinates patient navigator and other HSS curricular logistics. This institutional infrastructure commitment is necessary for program sustainability.

IMPLEMENTATION HISTORY AND STRATEGIES EMPLOYED

The CWRU SOM has a long-standing tradition of curricular innovation dating back to the 1910 Flexner Report.[8] In 2006, the SOM curriculum was redesigned in response to numerous drivers, such as a changing context of medicine and health systems (Fig. 5.1). The university track curriculum was designed to start with Block 1: Becoming A Doctor, which focuses on teaching elements of HSS, including public and population health and quality improvement.[9] In 2013, the Block 1 curriculum was further refined and redesigned into weeks, starting with population health, and then moving to determinants of health, health systems, and patient-centered care (Table 5.1). The basic science tools of caring for populations and communities are also featured in the block, including epidemiology and biostatistics, as well as the longitudinal theme of bioethics. The block includes large-group didactic sessions, small-group problem-based learning sessions, and team-based learning

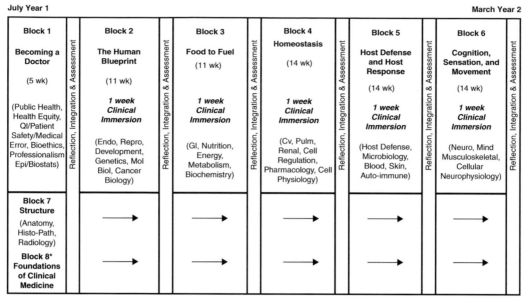

Fig. 5.1 Case Western Reserve University School of Medicine Preclinical Curriculum. (Adapted from Ornt DB, Aron DC, King NB, et al. Population medicine in a curricular revision at Case Western Reserve. *Acad Med.* 2008;83(4):327–331.)

exercises in population health, health systems, and climate change. The block also includes pandemic influenza and poverty simulations. Block 1 serves as the foundational HSS course, which is followed by a series of courses that weave a 4-year longitudinal HSS curricular thread throughout the undergraduate curriculum. At the CWRU SOM, all curricular blocks are managed by design teams that include students. There is also an overarching HSS design team that focuses on all elements of this curriculum through the undergraduate medical education experience.

First-year medical students consistently complete Block 1, activating and requesting experiential opportunities to further learn HSS and work as change agents during their journey through undergraduate medical education. Thus, in 2016, upon joining the AMA Accelerating Change in Medical Education Consortium and through guidance from colleagues at Penn State College of Medicine who had established a patient navigator program, an elective program in patient health system navigation was developed to provide a longitudinal HSS opportunity.[5]

In addition to the patient navigator program, we offer a range of community elective opportunities to first-year medical students upon completion of Block 1. These serve as supplemental opportunities beyond the standard curriculum and include patient navigator, an "aging in place" course, the student-run free clinic, and a

community-based interprofessional experience known as I-LEAP. Students are selected for these electives through an application process, which is necessary, as student demand is consistently higher than program capacity. During the application process, students rank desire for participation in the navigation program at the VA or NFP among other opportunities.

KEY ADVICE FOR FEASIBILITY AND SUSTAINABILITY

The intersection of value-added medical education innovations and HSS is critically important to adequately train the next generation of health professionals. Schools must emphasize HSS education across the medical education continuum in order to foster systems citizenship and train systems thinkers who are activated as change agents.[10]

The CWRU patient navigator experience highlights the importance of appropriate sequencing of HSS content to ensure a foundation prior to entering a community elective. The curricular journey through Block 1 prepares students to enter the PN elective with an HSS foundation that also enables students to appreciate the ways in which they provide value to the patient, health care team, and system. At CWRU, students do not always readily appreciate the

TABLE 5.1	Block 1 Curricular Overview					
	Weekly Theme	Problem-Based Learning Case	Unnatural Causes Episodes	Community Field Experiences	Team-Based Learning Exercise	Other Experiences
Week 1	Population Health		In Sickness and in Wealth; Not Just a Paycheck			Pandemic Influenza Simulation
Week 2	Determinants of Health	Toni Jackson: Determinants of Health	When the Bough Breaks; Place Matters	Determinants of Health/ Social Work	Population Health	Poverty Simulation
Week 3	Health Systems	Mr. Prince: Medical Error	Collateral Damage; Becoming American	Health Systems/ Safety Net	Global Health Systems Comparisons	Institute for Healthcare Improvement Open School Quality Improvement modules
Week 4	Patient-Centered Care	Mrs. Sanchez: Diabetes Mellitus	Bad Sugar	Chronic Conditions		
Week 5	"Bringing It All Together"	Jack Lee: Well Adult Care/ Addiction			Climate Change	

value they provide; thus, this is a focus of faculty mentorship and concretely reinforced in monthly meetings.

The commitment of CWRU SOM leadership to community health and HSS through public declarations of strategic priorities—as well as concrete commitments of faculty and staff protected time, as described previously—has been critical to initiation and maintenance of this program. Furthermore, long-standing formal partnerships with community organizations beyond traditional health system partners has been critical to placing students in meaningful patient navigator electives. In the CWRU patient navigator program, the partnerships with the Cleveland VA and NFP, both nationally recognized patient-centered medical homes with embedded CWRU faculty and an organizational commitment to allowing preclinical students EHR access and an equal place on an interprofessional team, have been critical to program success.

The main challenges in implementation and sustainment of the CWRU PN program center around capacity. While dedicated faculty and staff have been critical to

success, they also must balance this one elective serving up to 30 students per year with other responsibilities that serve the entire student body. Additionally, despite the HSS design team working to create a menu of HSS electives, the capacity of community sites to host students longitudinally remains limited, not enabling the entire class of nearly 200 students to participate. The balance of meaningful longitudinal value-added experiences is limited by capacity to host students in the current context of clinical care. It is perhaps in these challenges that further innovation in rethinking the intersection of HSS education and value-added roles will emerge.

CONCLUSION

The emerging field of HSS is ripe with opportunity to explore and innovate at the intersection with value-added roles in the context of rapidly changing health systems, particularly in the face of the COVID-19 pandemic. Programs such as patient navigator serve as early beacons of the possibilities that exist in redesigning health professions education to foster **equity** and relationship-grounded, whole-person care—ultimately leading to healthier individuals, healthier communitiesdical students partnered with newly arrived refugee and more equitable health systems.

REFERENCES

1. Leep Hunderfund AN, Starr SR, Dyrbye LN, et al. Value-added activities in medical education: a multisite survey of first- and second-year medical students' perceptions and factors influencing their potential engagement. *Acad Med.* 2018;93(10):1560–1568.
2. Skochelak SE, Hawkins RE, Lawson LE, Starr SR, Borkan JM, Gonzalo JD. *Health Systems Science.* Philadelphia: Elsevier; 2020.
3. Case Western Reserve University. First year students serve as patient navigators. *Medicus.* 2018. https://case.edu/medicine/sites/case.edu.medicine/files/2018-08/Medicus_Summer%20 2018.pdf. Accessed January 5, 2021.
4. Murphy B. As health navigators, students see value of team approach. 2018. https://www.ama-assn.org/education/accelerating-change-medical-education/health-navigators-students-see-value-team-approach. Published February 20, 2018. Accessed January 5, 2021.
5. Gonzalo JD, Haidet P, Papp KK, et al. Educating for the 21st-century health care system: an interdependent framework of basic, clinical and systems sciences. *Acad Med.* 2017;92(1):35–39.
6. Lockeman KS, Dow AW, DiasGrandos D, et al. Refinement of the IPEC Competency Self-Assessment Survey: results from a multi-institutional study. *J Interprof Care.* 30(6):726–731.
7. Dolansky MA, Moore SM, Palmieri PA, Singh MK. Development and validation of the Systems Thinking Scale. *J Gen Intern Med.* 2020;35(8):2314–2320.
8. Williams G. *Western Reserve's Experiment in Medical Education and Its Outcome.* New York: Oxford University Press; 1980.
9. Ornt DB, Aron DC, King NB, et al. Population medicine in a curricular revision at Case Western Reserve. *Acad Med.* 2008;83(4):327–331.
10. Gonzalo JD, Singh MK. Building Systems Citizenship in Health Professions Education: The Continued Call for Health Systems Science Curricula. https://psnet.ahrq.gov/perspective/building-systems-citizenship-health-professions-education-continued-call-health-systems. Published February 1, 2019. Accessed January 5, 2021.
11. Nutting PA, Goodwin MA, Flocke SA, Zyzanski SJ, Stange KC. Continuity of primary care: to whom does it matter and when? *Ann Fam Med.* 2003;1(3):149–155.
12. Etz RS, Zyzanski SJ, Gonzalez MM, Reves SR, O'Neal JP, Stange KC. A new comprehensive measure of high-value aspects of primary care. *Ann Fam Med.* 2019;17:221–230.
13. Long N, Wolpaw DR, Boothe D, et al. Contributions of health professions students to health system needs during the COVID-19 pandemic: potential strategies and process for medical schools. *Acad Med.* 2020. Online ahead of print. PMCID: PMC7375189.
14. Christ G, Dissell R. Cuyahoga County 'disease detectives,' CWRU medical students track coronavirus in one of Ohio's hotspots. *Cleveland Plain Dealer.* https://www.cleveland.com/business/2020/03/cuyahoga-county-disease-detectives-cwru-medical-students-track-coronavirus-in-one-of-ohios-hotspots.html. Published March 21, 2020. Accessed January 5, 2021.
15. School of Medicine students quickly ramp up to help manage crush of calls to local health centers. *The Daily.* https://thedaily.case.edu/school-of-medicine-students-quickly-ramp-up-to-help-manage-crush-of-calls-to-local-health-centers/. Published March 23, 2020. Accessed January 5, 2021.

FACULTY AND STUDENT REFLECTIONS

Program Vignettes: Student, Patient, and Community Partner Impact

Partnership With Newly Arrived Refugee Families at an FQHC

First-year medical students partnered with newly arrived refugee families and forged relationships with their partner families over the course of a year extending into the summer and the second year of medical school. They partnered with families who escaped war in Syria, Afghanistan, and Ethiopia, among other areas of the world. The following examples chronicle medical student navigators partnered with families facing serious behavioral and physical health issues while transitioning to a new country, culture, and language. Navigators embraced the notion of creating authentic trusting relationships by employing cultural humility and gaining the trust of their partner families. These students approached each family with kindness and attentiveness to their most pressing needs in order to eventually address health needs and promote well-being. Additionally, they seamlessly integrated themselves into primary care teams, becoming trusted among colleagues and even consistently documenting progress notes in the electronic health record (EHR).

In the first cohort of navigators, a first-year medical student accompanied a young mother to numerous oncology appointments and uncovered communication errors between providers that ultimately delayed treatment. He used this experience to advocate for EHR interoperability, noting, "If not me and now, then who and when?" This student, who later entered a career in primary care, noted in his second year of medical school that his patient navigator experience "taught me more about patient care than any series of lectures or other entity within the CWRU curriculum. I realized that I crave strong relationships with patients and want to help with their social issues, as well as their medical ones. I have gained a deep appreciation for the breadth and strength of the social determinants of health, as well as the shocking and unacceptable inadequacy of how health care is delivered in this country. I hope that I will soon get off of my chair and become active in changing these systems, so that we can truly both do no harm and provide each patient with the level of healing that he/she deserves."

In another example, two medical student navigators partnered with a mother and adult daughter from Afghanistan who experienced serious trauma as a result of war. While the mother had been dismissed by some physicians as having "somatic complaints," the navigators attended specialty and primary care appointments to articulate all of her concerns in the context of her past trauma, living situation, and profound social determinants of health. The students facilitated treatment for a bedbug infestation in the home, new health insurance when the woman and her daughter were disenrolled, and coordinated with the pharmacy when multiple medications were not filled due to insurance and communication errors. They also helped the family obtain clothing and food when those basic resources were scarce and advocated for transition to a new case manager and trauma therapist when they identified gaps in her care at one agency. They ultimately assisted the primary care physician in making the diagnosis of rheumatoid arthritis, leading to more effective systemic treatment options for pain control rather than continued dismissal as trauma-related somatic complaints. They accomplished all of this while using an interpreter to communicate in Dari. This family has repeatedly shared their gratitude for the role the navigators have played in this difficult transition to the US.

A different team of medical student navigators worked tirelessly in an advocacy role alongside a family from Syria with a young child who has a congenital anomaly resulting in tibial agenesis. The parents, who speak Arabic, did not want to proceed with amputation, but rather felt the best choice for their child was bilateral reconstruction that was not covered by insurance. The navigators advocated for this family's clinical options by obtaining imaging from Baltimore, which was completed at an earlier consult, and contacted a surgeon in Dubai (after exhausting all other options in the US in five states). They mailed the films to the surgeon in Dubai and communicated with him about how to make the reconstruction a reality for this child. They continued close communication with both parents using an interpreter and have also assisted the child's mother with diabetic education.

In a fourth example, a pair of students worked tirelessly coordinating care between primary care and specialists for a family from Ethiopia with two adult children who have severe cognitive and physical impairments. Their adult daughter's primary care physician identified that she had several years of biliary colic markedly impacting her eating patterns and daily function. The navigators worked to ensure that the family was able to obtain imaging and a surgical consult, as well as ultimately ensure that the surgery was successfully completed. They also advocated for a new psychiatry provider when the son was dismissed from specialty care after being told "nothing could be done for him" despite his parents being overwhelmed at times by his outbursts. The positive changes in care for both adult children were the result of their navigators' tireless advocacy and communication between multiple health care teams across three separate systems. Additionally, they worked to ensure that the mother was able to complete latent tuberculosis assessment and treatment as well as ensure that she had regular follow-up for severe asthma.

Finally, a fifth pair of students forged a beautiful relationship with a family of six from Syria with three children who were diagnosed with a life-threatening rare genetic anomaly affecting motor function. Two of the children are in wheelchairs and a third has muscular abnormalities at a young age. They worked to ensure that the many consultants and therapy appointments were coordinated, and that the family had their basic needs met, including helping when their wheelchair-accessible van was stolen and the oldest child was hit by a car while in his motorized wheelchair. The NFP primary care patient advocate has repeatedly expressed her gratitude for the work of the navigators and remarked how their care enabled far more services to be received than would have been possible without their advocacy. She wrote, "I have had the privilege to have been working closely with the Case students. Their willingness to assist patients in scheduling appointments and providing the care team with feedback about additional needs the patients have has been vital to patient care. This working relationship has been so helpful in my role as a patient advocate. I am very grateful for their support."

These remarkable medical students are change agents and systems citizens, bringing unparalleled value to the care of these families. They have shown the way for relationships and whole-person care to be realized in an increasingly commodity-driven health care system that incentivizes visits over time and longitudinal relationships.[11-13] Through practical experience, these students have learned the impact of social determinants of health and the need for physicians to be health systems champions in order to ensure better health for both individuals and communities. These navigation examples also demonstrate the extraordinary value that medical students bring to the health care system through their brilliant minds, incredible empathy, and drive to make the world a better place. These students have demonstrated that they bring tremendous value to patient care despite seemingly insurmountable social determinants, cultural and language differences, insurance limitations, and only a few months of medical school training before beginning this program.

VALUE-ADDED ROLES IN THE ERA OF COVID-19

As COVID-19 rapidly impacted the greater Cleveland community in early March 2020, health professions students were unable to continue in clinical and community rotations. As a result of the long-standing community relationships in the patient navigator program, a new telehealth rotation placed first-year through fourth-year medical and physician assistant students at the Cuyahoga County Board of Health (CCBH) and Neighborhood Family Practice (NFP), the federally qualified community health center (FQHC) patient navigator site, to serve in critical COVID-19 response roles.[14,15]

At NFP, students staffed a very busy call center, answering patient inquiries and communicating with the primary care teams. At CCBH, students joined the case interview and contact tracing teams, which created critically important capacity among rapidly expanding case numbers. A senior medical student, also a graduate of the patient navigator program, served as the student lead along with a CWRU faculty member who was also a patient navigator program lead and is embedded at the health department as the faculty population health liaison, training students in case interviewing, contact tracing, phone bank staffing, and response procedures for issuing isolation and quarantine letters. The students also worked closely with preventive medicine residents and local public health professionals, creating an interprofessional COVID-19 telehealth team serving the greater Cleveland community in a profoundly difficult time. Furthermore, the lead student in this response recorded videos and created extensive system maps that increased the efficiency of the response, while sharing her work with other medical students around the country to enable similar experiences. She ultimately created trainings for a team of contact tracers for the state of Ohio, sharing her on-the-ground COVID-19 and health systems expertise.

This timely example of pivoting to new, innovative value-added roles for health professions students demonstrates the power of creating the infrastructure and relationships with community partners that enable value-added roles for health professions students.[13] These students were prepared to serve their community in an evolving pandemic due to the robust health systems science curriculum in their early preclinical training, including a pandemic simulation, coupled with experiential health systems science learning, such as the patient navigator program.

6

Primary Care Quality Improvement: The University of North Carolina at Chapel Hill

Amy W. Shaheen, Shana Ratner, Kelly Bossenbroek Fedoriw, and Jan Lee Santos

LEARNING OBJECTIVES

1. Describe an example of a program of didactic and experiential learning in quality improvement methods.
2. Discuss key elements of context and program implementation that facilitate quality improvement education alongside quality improvement projects.
3. Identify opportunities for students to add value to a clinical setting through quality improvement efforts.
4. Explain the role of faculty in this novel quality improvement educational project.

OUTLINE

CHAPTER SUMMARY

In this chapter, we describe didactic and experiential learning for both students and faculty in quality improvement (QI) methods at the University of North Carolina at Chapel Hill. We describe our curriculum for early clinical learners in ambulatory care practices spread across our state and multiple health care systems. We share best practices for managing student concerns and faculty capacity for teaching QI. When relevant, we describe how to "shrink the change" so that others considering implementing an experiential QI curriculum do not feel overwhelmed.

INTRODUCTION

In 2014, when we initiated our current curriculum, medical students frequently complained about the lack of "good care" at their assigned primary care offices. Not uncommonly, a student would cite nonadherence with recommended guidelines or inefficient offices as reasons for their dissatisfaction. The students viewed these gaps as poor doctoring, not considering root causes. This care variation also created dissatisfaction as learners judged the physicians rather than partnering with them to find solutions. Students did not feel ownership for system improvements.

Despite this, we believed that students could bring significant insights and advantages to practices. Students encounter "bright spots" rotating from site to site that are potentially applicable to other settings. The students are facile with technology, nonthreatening to staff, and enthusiastic. They enjoy participating in crafting solutions and change ideas.

In order for students to share insights with physicians and be empowered to act, we had to create a curriculum that would make their ideas for system improvements a learning goal aligned with practice priorities. We had to change expectations for both students and physicians and prove this change would be valuable to leaders, systems, practices, physicians, patients, and students.

For the health of our patients and the sustainability of the system, our future physicians needed to understand how to improve systems of care.[1] While systems impact everything from our colon cancer screening rates to our own personal satisfaction, skilled individuals must ultimately drive the change. Building capacity for change in our future physician leaders required deliberate planning, teaching, and practice in QI methods.

Similar to the basic sciences and clinical sciences, deliberate practice in QI makes students better by applying learned skills.[2] Success and small failures in safe environments result in accelerated learning.[3] Unfortunately, medical schools do not traditionally reward failure as a learning tool. Failure on a basic science exam or failure in the clinical environment has serious implications for the student. However, that is not the case for QI projects.

Learning QI can be a relief and fun for students when properly incentivized and supported. Students are told to fail fast and learn what works. They are encouraged to watch for and learn from proximate reactions to changes in staff, physicians, and patients. For some, this is disconcerting and scary. In the mindset of "never fail," they may try to make changes independent of a team, leading to repeat failures. But failure should not be viewed as a lack of learning. Through purposeful reflection, students can gain insight into the complexity of systems, the nature of teams and leadership, and the difficulty of change. These failures and successes change student perspectives on what constitutes a good doctor or practice.

DESCRIPTION OF THE PROGRAM AT THE UNIVERSITY OF NORTH CAROLINA AT CHAPEL HILL

We began with small changes, grew expectations, partnered with essential stakeholders, and measured and shared our successes. We relied heavily on available resources and shared links to those curricular materials. We believe that any teacher can do the same if the teacher sets achievable goals, is willing to fail fast, and accept that the curriculum, the student, the faculty, the patient, or practice will never be perfect. Creating a QI curriculum is an iterative process apropos of the learning. Failure is to be expected, accepted, and remedied. Finally, the value of learning and applying QI in a real practice setting should be measured and shared. With these values in mind, we created an integrated curriculum culminating in a QI project during required outpatient clinical rotations. The curriculum is detailed in the Implementation History and Strategies Employed section of this chapter.

LEARNING GOALS

The learning goals for our curriculum are:
- Identify why you need to learn about QI.
- Discuss your role in a QI project.
- Learn how to develop a SMART (specific, measurable, achievable, relevant, and time bound) aim statement.
- Review the three tenets for the Model for Improvement.
- Learn the fundamentals of a driver diagram.
- Review course expectations for QI and trimester timeline.

TECHNIQUES TO ASSESS LEARNERS

Curricular learning goals and assessments should align. For example, if the learning goal of a QI curriculum is to understand QI terms, then a multiple-choice test might suffice. To assess application of that knowledge to a simulated case, the modified Quality Improvement Knowledge Application Tool (QIKAT) may suffice.[4] When doing experiential QI learning, the summative assessments and practice needs should align.

Engagement with a QI project provides students with an opportunity to apply concepts and skills learned during the didactic and self-directed learning components of the curriculum. Students are supported by designated clinical staff and course faculty to ensure that time and effort contribute to both student and clinic improvement goals. The students collaborate with the clinic's staff and/or clinicians to identify an area of improvement, use a template for project management, and perform three Plan-Do-Study-Act (PDSA) cycles. Students receive assistance with project design, team formation, data collection, and QI poster creation from faculty as well as clinical QI leads or coaches during the 16 weeks. We created several documents to serve as resources and guides that allow student projects to flow smoothly. These include a modified A3 template (a Lean Six Sigma one-page project management tool),[5] a poster template, and a poster grading form. A QI weekly schedule containing learning objectives, assignments, tasks to be completed, and proposed deadlines for QI deliverables is useful in providing a structured timeline.

In early iterations of the curriculum and because students were creating real projects, we chose to use the QI proposal assessment tool, or QIPAT, to evaluate one PDSA of the student's choice.[6] However, because one PDSA did not represent the sum of a student's work, we ultimately chose to use an end-of-project poster for evaluation. We created a grading rubric to reward iteration, learning, poster appearance, and communication. The poster counts for 3% of a student's grade.

The poster grading rubric was distributed to students, preceptors, and clinical QI coaches to use as a guide in the creation of their posters. Having the rubric ahead of time helps students align their projects and posters to the specific QI project requirements and makes the grading transparent. In addition, QI poster exemplars are provided on our course website to standardize poster appearance and organization of content. The examples are good for helping students appropriately scope their projects as well.

Posters are graded by core faculty and local QI experts using a rubric with a possible 15 points (Fig. 6.1). Students are also awarded course credit for completion of the

	Criteria	Max # Points	Points Given
TITLE	Reflects interventions and goals (or outcomes)	1	
BACKGROUND	Clearly stated, explains why this is an important problem	1	
AIM STATEMENT	Can you easily identify an AIM-statement?	1	
	Is this a SMART aim (Specific, Measurable, Achievable, Relevant, Timely)	1	
METHODS	SETTING was adequately described (clinic/practice size and type, patient population, # of providers)	1	
	PROCESS was explained such that another clinic could replicate it (planning/baseline data, intervention(s), team members and individual roles etc)	1	
	DATA COLLECTION was clearly outlined (process vs outcome measures, how data was collected and/or analyzed)	1	
	Were **at least** 3 specific PDSAs/changes highlighted?	1	
RESULTS	The results were easy to understand	1	
	Results clearly showed how interventions impacted data? (Ex: graphs/charts, before and after data, and/or statistical measures) **If applicable** – There is a graph to accurately represent improvements/changes over time (Ex: run chart, bar graphs)	**2 total**	
CONCLUSION	Reasonable, logical conclusion from results	1	
	Limitations of study/results described	1	
	Future directions or follow-up projects identified	1	
GENERAL	Poster is well organized, well edited and easy to read	1	
TOTAL		15	

Maximum Points = 15, 1/2 points are allowed for partial credit

Did this project involve at least 3 clearly identifiable PDSAs.   YES/NO
Is this the BEST poster you graded (choose only 1)   YES/NO

Fig. 6.1 QI Poster Grading Rubric.

assigned Institute for Healthcare Improvement (IHI)[7] modules and A3 project management tool. The QI component is worth 5% of the students' final grade in the course.

The culmination of the curriculum is the QI Poster Dinner, a celebratory dinner held at the end of the 16 weeks where each student's poster is displayed and evaluated. Holding the dinner during week 15 generally leaves enough time for studying for any final exams the following week. Students, their families, preceptors, clinic staff, QI coaches, faculty, and school of medicine leaders are all encouraged to attend the 2-hour dinner, held in a nearby banquet hall. The celebratory environment encourages discussions among all attendees as they mingle and view the posters. Each attendee (including adult family members) is assigned six to eight posters to rate at the start of the session. We do this because we feel that a good QI project should be understandable by anyone, including patients or families. At the end of the evening, all scores are tallied, and $25 gift cards are given to first-, second-, and third-place posters. This score does not affect the students' grade, but the gift cards are a fun incentive. This event provides an opportunity to learn about the successes and challenges of other clinic sites, discuss new trends and approaches in solving problems, network with other individuals involved in QI, and learn best practices in teaching and integrating learners into the clinic.

After the dinner, student posters are displayed in the practices in which they worked. This is a way of giving back to the staff, physicians, and patients who participated in the project. The posters also serve as a hand-off tool to the next student, who is encouraged to review the poster if asked to work on the same practice measure.

Finally, for course directors beginning an experiential QI curriculum, the course duration will dictate the assignments and whether a project management tool is necessary. Prior to 2016, we had an ambulatory 4-week internal medicine course that required students to do one PDSA cycle that was graded with the QIPAT. As we lengthened the course from 4 to 6 and now 16 weeks, we increased the number of PDSA cycles that a student must do in the practice. Currently, we require a minimum of three PDSAs. Most students do more than required, anxious for improvement. Completion of the A3 project management tool is a mandatory assignment for which students receive 1% of their grades. The other 1% of a student's grade comes from completion of the required IHI modules, which we track centrally.

EVALUATION PROCEDURES

Curricula can be evaluated using many Kirkpatrick levels.[8] We were able to measure student satisfaction through usual year-end evaluations, student application of knowledge (behavior change) with the QIPAT, and patient outcomes via the practice capacity for students and practice dashboards.

Student Satisfaction

After the preclinical phase of the curriculum, we administered an evaluation of course content for the entire 18 months to the medical students. Students have had brief exposure to the QI content at this point. Another program evaluation is administered at the end of medical school, which is approximately a year after experiencing the QI curriculum. Students responded to questions using rating scales for each item. We would recommend that course directors considering an experiential QI curriculum look at current evaluation forms and add questions to existing forms if needed. The curriculum phase evaluation questions that follow already existed, and we used these retrospectively. We would encourage course directors to adapt current surveys to measure student satisfaction prior to curriculum change.

For our first evaluation, medical students responded to the following prompt: "Please rate how familiar overall you are with the examples of the terms and concepts: Quality Improvement and safety; e.g., PDSA; Aim statement; Institutional reporting systems for near misses; Root cause analysis; Triple Aim." Ratings were from 1 = poor to 5 = excellent. Preclinical medical school classes from 2017 to 2019 rated this prompt as 2.6 (n = 158), 2.8 (n = 158), and 2.9 (n = 136), respectively.

A second question asked how confident students were in their current ability to perform specified activities at the beginning of clinical rotations: "Use standard approaches and measures of quality improvement to enhance patient care such as assessing a clinic's adherence to national clinical guidelines and its measured patient satisfaction levels." Ratings were from 1 = not at all confident to 5 = very confident. Medical school classes from 2017 to 2019 rated this prompt as 2.8 (n = 159), 2.9 (n = 156), and 3.2 (n =133), respectively.

On the end of the medical school program evaluation, students again responded to the prompt: "Please rate how familiar overall you are with the examples of the terms and concepts: Quality Improvement and safety; e.g., PDSA; Aim statement; Institutional reporting systems for near misses; Root cause analysis; Triple Aim." Medical school classes from 2017 to 2019 rated this prompt as 3.8 (n = 146), 3.9 (n = 131), and 3.7 (n = 141), respectively.

While these questions are fundamentally different and do not constitute a true pre/post-assessment, they were pedagogically sound. They asked questions pertinent to the teaching and learning expectations of the students. Based on the responses, we felt confident that our curriculum was meeting our goals.

Student Behavior Change

In order to assess students' application of QI methods, we chose to evaluate their performance developing a QI project plan with the QIPAT. Students received formative feedback by another student on the first draft of their PDSA cycle using QIPAT.[6] One of three faculty members used the QIPAT to provide a second round of formative feedback (including comments) on the first PDSA by week 8 of the course for all students. We did not record scores, as this was formative feedback. Course directors considering programmatic evaluation should consider using this tool to monitor student progress.

Course directors and QI experts also evaluated the posters. While we did not use the QIPAT for programmatic evaluation, we feel that this could be a possibility for others to consider.

Preceptor Engagement

Prior to the implementation of this innovation, we faced challenges identifying preceptors willing to teach students.[9–11] One of the measures we sought to improve was willingness of preceptors to accept student clinical placements. With the new longitudinal curricular format and inclusion of the QI requirement in March of 2016, the number of potential student placements with preceptors increased from 16 to 64. The number of placements in community health clinics increased from 4 to 12, and the university-affiliated practice placements increased from 2 to 20. The number of private clinic placements increased from 10 to 30 training sites. We currently have a total of 75 pediatric, family medicine, and internal medicine faculty involved; 45 is the maximum number of placements needed per trimester, meaning we have a net surplus.

Prior efforts by the school of medicine leadership to increase capacity for clinical preceptors had not been successful. Course directors heard from a variety of sources (imbedded coaches, practice and care managers, and health system leaders) that the QI curriculum helped practices and that leadership wanted students placed in as many practices as they could. Highly performing or improving practices likely reflected well on those same leaders. These leaders consequently asked more practices and providers to host students.

Practice Outcomes

Using clinical quality metrics from monthly dashboards at the university and Chapel Hill clinics, projects were aligned to institutional or systems priorities for QI. This allowed us to compare dashboard metrics with metrics on which students worked. Private practice quality dashboards were unavailable; however, we were able to categorize projects to determine care priorities for their practices.

Student projects and alignment with practice or institutional measures included but were not limited to diabetes management, colorectal cancer screening, and mental health screening.[12] The top choices for projects in private practices included diabetes at 17.3% (9/52), mental health at 19.2% (10/52), and opioid monitoring at 13.5% (7/52).

We created mechanisms for local dissemination and encouraged regional and national dissemination of student projects. First, we established the aforementioned poster dinner at the end of each block. This event ensured that all students had the opportunity to present their work at least once.

Dozens of students have also presented their work to our statewide University of North Carolina (UNC) Primary Care Improvement Collaborative (PCIC). Both UNC faculty practices and UNC hospital-owned practices participate in the collaborative. Students have shared their PDSAs and lessons learned with coaches and team members from 63 other practices across the state. Students with particularly impactful projects are strongly encouraged to present their work to facilitate spread.

One Community-Based Longitudinal Care (CBLC) student, for example, helped make the PCIC quality metrics more tangible by showing that how we displayed the data could be improved. Prior to his intervention, all measures were shown simply as percentage achieved—for example, percent of patients with a mammogram in the last year. Through an iterative process, this student was able to show that providers did not know how to interact with or respond to that number. Providers described feeling helpless to change it. Therefore, he created a "number of patients to goal" and found that providers responded much more positively to that number. When he showed the number of patients to vaccinate out of 30 to reach the pneumonia vaccine goal, he found providers much more amenable to his changes. The student shared this proposed change at the PCIC operations meeting, where multiple other clinics reported that this would be helpful in change management for their clinics. The overall PCIC dashboard was then adjusted to include this for all metrics and all clinics. This change has been sustained. At Piedmont Health Services (PHS), a similar improvement collaborative for their 10 practice sites has been established. Students present their results at the collaborative meeting, stimulating the spread of ideas.

Many students also submitted abstracts to regional and national meetings. Our students have displayed posters, have given oral presentations, and received recognitions locally, regionally, and nationally. There have been numerous publications related to student QI projects (a list can be found at https://www.med.unc.edu/ihqi/programs/medical-student-scholarly-concentration/student-abstracts-1/). In addition to student dissemination, the rotation leaders have disseminated their learnings from student experiences in QI through national presentations and manuscripts.[2,12]

Advanced Learners

In parallel to the development of the CBLC QI curriculum, an advanced learner course was developed. This elective course is available to fourth-year medical students and is an extracurricular scholarly concentration in QI called Clinical Leaders in Quality and Safety. Students are paired with an expert in QI on a system-wide QI project. Students participate in didactic sessions with QI system leaders. We consider participation in this scholarly concentration a measure of early learner success. To date, 36 medical students have participated in this fourth-year elective.

RESOURCES NEEDED

The resources necessary for the curriculum include didactic time, faculty time, and the financial support for printing posters and providing the poster dinner. The didactic time has been outlined in other sections. Faculty time includes one core faculty member to lead the didactic sessions as well as provide support to students, practices, and

QI coaches as students work on their projects. Many of our clinics have their own QI coaches or local QI experts, but not all. Support for those students placed at a clinic without an expert include outreach and faculty office hours for students who want advice or help on their projects. Any student can attend these sessions, but they are particularly helpful for students without local QI expertise. Printing the posters for 45 students costs approximately $1,100. The dinner is held three times a year for about $3,000 for each event. The total yearly cost, which does not include faculty time, is $12,300.

IMPLEMENTATION HISTORY AND STRATEGIES EMPLOYED

Curriculum

The UNC School of Medicine curriculum is divided into three phases: foundation phase, application phase, and individualization phase (Fig. 6.2). The foundation phase integrates basic sciences, early clinical experiences, organ systems, and social and health system sciences (SHSS) over a period of 17 months. The SHSS curriculum in the first 17 months lays the foundation for the experiential QI learning in the application phase. The curriculum covers professional identity formation, medical ethics, health care systems, advocacy, leadership, teamwork, change management, and social determinants of health.

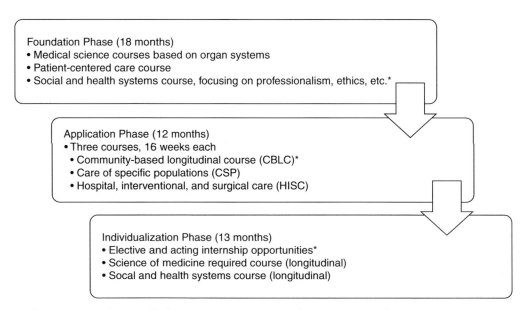

Foundation Phase (18 months)
• Medical science courses based on organ systems
• Patient-centered care course
• Social and health systems course, focusing on professionalism, ethics, etc.*

Application Phase (12 months)
• Three courses, 16 weeks each
  • Community-based longitudinal course (CBLC)*
  • Care of specific populations (CSP)
  • Hospital, interventional, and surgical care (HISC)

Individualization Phase (13 months)
• Elective and acting internship opportunities*
• Science of medicine required course (longitudinal)
• Socal and health systems course (longitudinal)

*Indicates course where quality improvement and patient safety are addressed·

Fig. 6.2 School of Medicine Curriculum Structure.

The application phase begins in March of the students' second year and consists of three 16-week trimesters named CBLC, Hospital, Interventional and Surgical Care, and Care of Specific Populations. Our experiential QI curriculum was strategically placed in the outpatient medicine course, CBLC. The third phase of the curriculum, individualization phase, is 15 months of electives, research opportunities, and acting internships. In this chapter, we discuss the experiential QI curriculum for early clinical learners during the CBLC course.

The QI curriculum integrated into the 16-week CBLC course combines didactic, experiential, and self-directed learning to help students understand QI methodologies and population health concepts while engaging in a meaningful QI project. The didactic component includes four classroom sessions scheduled throughout the 16-week course (Fig. 6.3). During these sessions, the students wrestle with the need to improve health care delivery, become familiar with QI methodologies, and begin to use tools such as driver diagrams and process maps. Students practice creating SMART aim statements as well as PDSA cycles, and get peer and faculty feedback during highly interactive sessions. During later sessions, we work on graphical representation of data. In the last session, the students discuss the social determinants of health (SDOH) and variation in data due to SDOH, the impact of their QI efforts in decreasing that variation, and advocacy for decreasing variation due to SDOH.

The self-directed learning component of the curriculum requires completion of 7 web-based IHI[7] modules during the first 6 weeks of the curriculum. The IHI modules are free and available online and were chosen based on their alignment with student learning objectives. The ability to track module completion is available to course directors for a small fee. The students complete IHI basic certificate modules QI 101 to 105, the Triple Aim, and the Patient- and Family-Centered Care modules. The basic certificate is then completed during their fourth-year SHSS course. Other self-directed assignments completed online via an educational software platform include developing a SMART AIM statement, identifying practice team members and mentors, completing a QI project that aligns with practice needs or measures, and recording change ideas and results on a modified A3 project management tool.[5]

Faculty Development

Students in the CBLC course have been placed in a wide variety of practice types, including faculty, hospital-owned, private, and community health practices. The faculty practices, both family medicine and internal medicine, serve over 25,000 patients at the main university campus. Students provide medical, nutrition, and behavioral health services. The faculty practices host approximately 10 students per block. The hospital-owned practices serve more than 100,000 patients over 5 counties. They offer medical

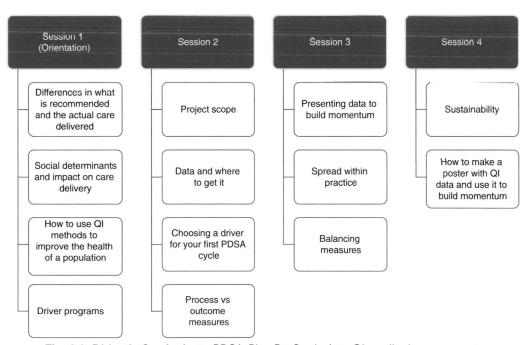

Fig. 6.3 Didactic Curriculum. *PDSA*, Plan-Do-Study-Act; *QI*, quality improvement.

services and have access to behavioral health and nutrition services within their network. The hospital-owned practices host approximately 10 to 12 students per block. Private practices offer the most variety in size and services. Some are multispecialty practices. Some are solo physicians, serving primarily insured patients. Services offered to patients vary. Office staff in private practices range from dozens to as few as four. Private practices host approximately six to eight students per block. The community health clinic, PHS, is a federally qualified health center (FQHC) with 10 community health centers and 2 senior care sites that provide medical, dental, pharmaceutical, behavioral health, nutrition, and women, infant, and children services to approximately 43,000 patients. PHS hosts 10 to 12 UNC CBLC students every block.

We found quite a bit of variability in the QI knowledge of the preceptors. At the onset of this program, preceptors did not feel prepared to mentor the students in a QI project based on their own perceived lack of knowledge and skills in QI. Therefore, preceptors were trained in QI using a variety of methods, such as co-learning, self-directed learning, didactics, and sharing of best practices. We began the QI improvement faculty curriculum with co-learning. We paired faculty development with student education and repeated a two-session faculty curriculum during faculty-student dinners three times in the first year of the curriculum. We had over 40 faculty participate in at least 2 dinner sessions our first year.

For those who were unable to attend the co-learning curriculum in the first year, we now encourage self-directed learning and have created a repository of materials through which faculty preceptors can learn QI concepts and aid in project development, implementation, and sustainability. There are three short videos available from UNC's web page dedicated to faculty teaching skills (https://www.med.unc.edu/teachingskills/). Topics include "Getting Started on your QI project," "PDSAs 101," and a "QI case study." The "Getting Started" video includes information on setting expectations with students; project selection, including topic and scope; QI versus research; data security; access to data in the electronic health record (EHR); and how to time and keep up with the project. PDSA 101 explains the concept of the PDSA cycle and provides multiple examples of how students might carry out these cycles in a clinic setting. The "QI case study" walks through one successful project from beginning to end.

Since the first year of the curriculum, we have periodically reintroduced the videos at the end-of-course poster sessions so that any new faculty can familiarize themselves with the concepts. While these videos have been available since 2017, we have only tracked the

site usage data since 2019. There were 83 views of the QI faculty development videos in 2019.

We also provide links to a publicly available website for QI resources in our "introduction to the new student" emails. These include QI project preceptor expectations, expected project timelines, templates for driver diagrams, AIM statements, PDSA cycles, and a modified A3.

After the first year of implementing our QI curriculum, we decreased our faculty development dinner sessions from six to three a year in response to available resources and the risk of overburdening preceptors. Rather than co-learning, we offer direct instruction on topics in clinical teaching and QI at a poster session dinner three times a year. After poster review and the dinner, a UNC faculty member or course director gives a short didactic on common QI concepts. Preceptors and students then discuss and attempt to apply these ideas to their current projects. For instance, we teach about how to create a driver diagram. Students and preceptors then build a driver diagram. Resources available to preceptors are widely shared at this session. The initial faculty development dinners occurred at week 4 and week 8. When we moved to one dinner per trimester at the end of the rotation, the table discussions became more reflective on lessons learned, how to address additional drivers, or maintain sustainability.

We also found that the dinner and poster sessions are great tools for shared learning. At the dinner, faculty evaluate posters of students from other sites, and faculty report that some of their best learning comes from evaluating those posters. Via the posters, preceptors can see how others tackled problems, scoped the problem for a student, displayed data, and created sustainable processes. In recognition of the value of the poster session, practice and system leaders attend the sessions and encourage their preceptors to attend.

Preceptors at PHS (the FQHC that hosts many students), UNC Health Care System (HCS) employed physicians and coaches, and UNC academic faculty have the opportunity to network during these dinners. These interactions have been valuable in creating trust among various participants in our health care system. Most of the practices engaged with our students have now joined our clinically integrated network. The student projects and celebratory dinners have offered an opportunity for demonstrating the value of an academic medical center to an entire community of physicians and patients and vice versa.

Implementation

At UNC School of Medicine, we have three large and distinct systems that teach the majority of our students—UNC Faculty Physicians, physicians employed by the UNC Health Care System, and the community health center, PHS. These large practices have all designated staff to provide guidance, resources, and support to students as they complete their QI projects, recognizing the return on investment in the students. The designated staff have duties already aligned with practice QI needs and view the students as valuable resources for meeting their own goals.

For example, at PHS, where 12 students are placed across 6 sites, the core QI team consists of a corporate QI coach, who oversees all practice QI work; a clinical preceptor, who provides onsite guidance and modifications to project design and/or PDSA cycles; and a medical education project manager, who monitors the student clinical schedule and designates time in the schedule for students to work on QI projects. On average, the corporate QI coach, clinical preceptor, and medical education project manager provide a total of 3 to 5 hours of QI project support per student each trimester. This ensures that students have designated sources of support from all levels of PHS to complete their rotations and projects as smoothly as possible.

The corporate QI coach, with input from PHS senior leadership, plans and designs projects aligned with current PHS goals. Projects are designed to simultaneously or sequentially tackle different drivers of the same metric throughout a given year. At the beginning of each rotation, the corporate QI coach provides data and descriptions for potential projects from which the students can choose. This coach also facilitates monthly check-ins, assists with poster creation using a UNC-provided rubric and record, catalogues projects, and disseminates results to the organization. For example, during one block, four students at one site simultaneously worked on different drivers to improve colon cancer screening. The lessons learned from that project informed change ideas for other clinical sites.

Any core team member can serve as the primary QI preceptor, engage and mobilize additional PHS staff to contribute as a process owner or subject matter expert, or provide help in data collection, extraction, and analysis. It is common for a student to have three to four PHS staff contribute significantly to a project.

During the first year of the QI curriculum at PHS, there was a significant amount of communication between students and the corporate QI coaches throughout the project. However, with faculty gaining familiarity with QI, project scope, expectations of students, and improved early communication, most of the discussion now happens during the first week of the block, improving efficiency for all.

At UNC HCS–owned practices, a QI coaching model already existed. These coaches are paid by the UNC HCS and are facilitators for change, visiting practices an average of 20 minutes a month and following up by email or phone as needed. The coaches work with practices, discuss change ideas, teach process owners how to access relevant data in the EHR, and share successful changes from other practices.

We felt the QI coaches would be good partners for students, and they easily agreed. QI coaches meet the students assigned to their practices at orientation. Coaches plan for high-yield student projects and serve as advocates for students in practices. The coaches are available to students to discuss barriers and solutions by email or in person. One coach has been very instrumental in setting timelines and creating the project management tool, the modified A3 template.[5] Recognizing that the language on a traditional A3 was foreign to students, the coach changed the A3 tool to reflect what students were actually doing, and the modified A3 became a class assignment. Due to student engagement in QI, the UNC HCS–owned practices have transformed from unwilling hosts of students to staunch supporters. Leaders from the UNC HCS and coaches regularly participate in our QI poster dinners. Leaders encourage physicians, nurses, and front desk staff to engage with student projects.

The UNC faculty practices also have staff designated for QI initiatives. These staff get data for students and grant them access to a secure server for patient data. Leaders in the UNC faculty practices prospectively consider measures needing improvement and designate mentors and team members for each student. Initially, the QI mentors and the clinical preceptors were not the same person, but we quickly realized that this led to confusion for the students. If a student has more than one clinical preceptor, we assign at least one mentor with QI experience. Rather than assign a QI project to a student, we assign the project to the mentor who then works with the assigned student to create drivers appropriately scoped for a student to tackle.

A course director considering implementing QI projects as part of a clinical course should actively seek out similar partners who can provide on-site support. Lack of partners should not preclude development of an experiential curriculum. Partnerships began at different times in the curriculum. Many of our private practices, where up to a fourth of our students are placed, do not have experienced QI staff or providers.

For all students, we offer QI office hours. The use of office hours is strongly encouraged for students at private practices. We offer 2 to 3 hours of walk-in or telephone help each trimester. Students who do not have dedicated staff for QI work are encouraged to come to office hours to help them scope the project, overcome hurdles to data acquisition, identify appropriate team members, and ensure that they are able to complete assignments. Students at these practices perform similarly to students at highly supported practices. Student projects at private practices have won recognitions at the poster dinner and have even been published.

In summary, use local resources when available and offer flexible support to those without those resources. Course directors should also identify and partner with those resources in an effort to meet local needs. Over time, local staff will gravitate to students if student improvements align with their own job descriptions.

Projects

When considering a QI project for a learner, it is important to consider learning goals, learner skill level, project duration, and the project sponsor. Learning goals should explicitly focus on understanding and attaining QI concepts and skills.[13] A number of learning theories have helped inform our understanding of experiential learning. Take-home points for successful experiential learning in QI include the importance of alignment with the dominant force (the motivations of clinical practices), consideration of the social context (faculty, staff), and the role of the student (acting as a negotiator for better processes or process ownership rather than a process participant). Thus, the best projects align with clinical measures, partner learners with the right team members and faculty sponsors, and focus on process changes. Course directors should emphasize the learning goals with students and explain that, once mastered, these goals could be applied to projects aligning with the learner's interests.

Student skill level and scope of project should match. Johnson et al. describe well what we learned as we implemented our curriculum.[14] Early learners should work to improve or develop new processes for a small team. These processes should ideally be relevant to their studies. This requires interactions with team members, iteration, and leadership skill development. A learner should read background information to inform the process. For example, a student might read the blood pressure guidelines and learn how to properly check a blood pressure before embarking on a project to improve blood pressure control for patients of a physician-nurse team. In this scenario, the student may work with a nurse on when and how to recheck a blood pressure, where to document repeat blood pressures, or when to notify the physician about the need for repeat blood pressures. In this situation, the student works on the process but is not the one responsible for the repeat blood pressures. In this way, a change is sustainable. In another example, a student working to improve outreach efforts on colon cancer screening would be encouraged to read about colon cancer screening modalities and then could work to improve processes for nurses handing

out stool cards. One of our students taught nurses how to do fecal immunochemical tests (FIT) during lunch using chocolate pudding. She then worked to improve the nurse process of identifying patients due for FIT tests. The focus on process allows for long-term sustainability in anticipation of learners eventually leaving the clinical environment.

The duration of the project will impact the choice and scope of the project.[14] Short-duration projects (< 1 month) are best aligned with one team. As the duration increases, more teams, physicians, or units can be engaged. Our curriculum stresses "getting to one" successful process early in the rotation. For example, a student improving a process where a nurse appropriately rechecks a high first blood pressure would be a success. The aim for this day's PDSA would be "have the team nurse appropriately repeat blood pressure in response to a high reading." Once that has occurred, then the intervention can be expanded, or the student learns what did not work and can remedy it quickly. Emphasize the first successful process or PDSA over 1 to 2 days.

Project leaders for early learners should be their assigned clinical preceptor to improve daily communication of successes and failures. Projects should improve processes that directly impact the preceptor and patients seen by the preceptor team. Failures in processes, such as not rechecking a blood pressure or missing a vaccine that had been flagged, should be researched immediately by the student to see why the proposed process failed in order to make adjustments. One student wanted to implement a questionnaire for patients with chronic obstructive pulmonary disease. She worked with front desk staff to prospectively identify patients and share that information with the nurses. Within one day she was able to see whether a nurse could respond to a shared comment in the EHR and hand out a questionnaire. When it did not happen as planned, the preceptor asked her to research why not and modify the next PDSA cycle.

Examples of projects at private practices include one student in a pediatric practice who worked to increase the screening for adverse childhood events. She documented improvement by counting the number of forms collected recording the adverse childhood events. The student was so encouraged by her success that, during her fourth year of medical school, she focused a scholarly concentration project at the same practice. During that time, she developed resources and strategies for responding to positive screens in patients and caregivers. Another student in a private practice worked to increase the use of masks for patients with respiratory symptoms. Working with faculty during the QI office hours, we discovered the importance of this to the practice (the whole practice was forced to shut down during a flu outbreak) and helped develop a driver diagram that included sustainable changes that would positively impact the practice. Her measure became the number of masks removed from the mask supply box daily. Her changes were sustainable, including patient education, placement of masks, and identification of a champion to continue to measure adherence to the process.

KEY ADVICE FOR FEASIBILITY AND SUSTAINABILITY

The UNC School of Medicine Education Committee provides governance over the entire medical degree curriculum and has established competencies that are mapped to each course over the 4-year curriculum. The health systems science competency states: "Students must demonstrate an awareness of and responsiveness to the larger system of health care and demonstrate the skills needed to improve the health of specific clinical populations." In addition, the Liaison Committee on Medical Education has a standard focused on self-directed and lifelong learning (Element 6.3), with the expectation that medical students begin to learn principles of QI and patient safety.

Prior to implementing our curriculum, most QI education happened in the preclinical years, isolated from clinical application. The preclinical component is "pre-work" that sets the stage for students to engage more fully with the QI concepts during their clinical years. Much like trying to learn how to ride a bike without the actual bike, students were participating in thoughtful discussions about medical errors, screening rates, and population health without actually putting these ideas into practice. The Education Committee endorsed experiential learning of health systems education, including QI. Through discussions with course leaders, appropriate curricular space was identified.

Therefore, under the direction of the School of Medicine Education Committee, this experiential curriculum was developed and supported. We encourage others considering a similar curriculum to obtain endorsement from their governing committees. This encourages continual improvement and responsiveness of school of medicine leadership when course directors encounter barriers.

The most important aspects to sustainability of a QI project are the alignment of project goals with practice goals and the recognition and use of students as facilitators for improvement rather than process owners. These two concepts must be linked. A student will not be able to facilitate change and identify process owners unless the initiative has a project sponsor and team members that align to practice priorities. Once aligned, team members are motivated to help a student make improvements. Students can observe processes and work to improve those processes among team members. Students may initially insert themselves to better understand the process and learn what does or does not work before transitioning the role to another team member. However, for long-term sustainability, the process role must ultimately shift to another team member.

For example, one trimester a student worked to understand the process of obtaining external results for diabetic eye exams. The student obtained multiple eye exams herself but used the learning to create a process map for another staff member to ultimately assume. Once the process was clear, she worked to educate the new process owner on the refined process.

Sustainability of the process is necessary but sustainability of practice buy-in for QI is also important. Practices celebrate student achievements regardless of results or outcomes. We encourage posters to be hung in practices to include recognition of all team members. Practice-wide announcements are made when students win an award for their work. Student presentations to senior leadership help maintain leadership support. At PHS, an annual report includes student names, pictures, biographies, and project results. A quarterly newsletter is emailed to all faculty and includes attachments of the best posters from the celebratory dinner. In summary, to ensure sustainability, align with practices, encourage facilitation of process change, and celebrate success to keep process owners and practices engaged.

CONCLUSION

QI curriculum benefits students, practices, health care systems, and patients. Course directors can create interdisciplinary experiential learning using many existing resources. Partnerships with health care systems increase capacity for learners. Systems benefit from additional resources and providers learn valuable skills with learners.

ACKNOWLEDGMENTS

The authors would like to recognize the contributions of Cristin Colford, MD, UNC Department of Medicine; Ronni Booth, UNC Health; Lynne Fiscus, MD, MPH, UNC Health; Nicole Chandler, MD, Cone Health Medical Group; Karina Whelan, MD, UNC Department of Medicine, and all of the providers from UNC Health and PHS as well as the quality coaches!

STUDENT REFLECTIONS

During my family medicine rotation in rural North Carolina, I had the opportunity to design and implement a QI project. After meeting with clinic staff to assess their needs and priorities, I focused my project on increasing hepatitis C screening rates. The project aimed to raise awareness and utilization of a new tool in the EHR, which displayed all appropriate screenings for each patient. After my rotation ended, another medical student built on this project by adding patient educational flyers about hepatitis C screening in the clinic. Together, we wrote a manuscript about the results, strengths, and limitations of our QI project, which was accepted for publication in the *Journal for Healthcare Quality*.

Melissa Klein, MPH
MD Candidate, UNC School of Medicine

The CBLC quality improvement project served as the capstone for my family medicine experience. I was naïve to the importance of QI work. With the tools I was given through a combination of in-person lectures and online modules, I was able to pinpoint which outcomes within our clinic contributed to the distribution of "quality care" to conduct a needs assessment focusing on areas for improvement. I found myself personally invested not only in the efficacy of our intervention but if patients were perceiving a difference in the quality of their care. The QI project not only introduced me to the practical difficulties of providing care in a federally qualified health center but brought me closer to my patients by encouraging me to examine the intricacies of each clinic visit from their perspective.

Lauren Catterall
MD Candidate, UNC School of Medicine

REFERENCES

1. Gonzalo JD, Caverzagie KJ, Hawkins RE, Lawson L, Wolpaw DR, Chang A. Concerns and responses for integrating health systems science into medical education. *Acad Med.* 2018;93(6):843–849.
2. Shaheen AW, Bossenbroek Fedoriw K, Khachaturyan S, et al. Students adding value: improving patient care measures while learning valuable population health skills. *Am J Med Qual.* 2019:1–9. https://doi.org/10.1177/1062860619845482.
3. Klasen JM, Lingard LA. Allowing failure for educational purposes in postgraduate clinical training: a narrative review. *Med Teach.* 2019;41(11):1263–1269.
4. Singh MK, Ogrinc G, Cox KR, et al. The quality improvement knowledge application tool revised (QIKAT-R). *Acad Med.* 2014;89(10):1386–1391.
5. Eby K. Free Lean Six Sigma Templates. https://www.smartsheet.com/free-lean-six-sigma-templates. Published June 12, 2017. Accessed 14.12.20.
6. Leenstra JL, Beckman TJ, Reed DA, et al. Validation of a method for assessing resident physicians' quality improvement proposals. *J Gen Int Med.* 2007;22(9):1330–1334. https://doi.org/10.1007/s11606-007-0260-y.
7. Institute for Healthcare Improvement. IHI Open School Online Courses. http://www.ihi.org/education/IHIOpenSchool/Courses/Pages/OpenSchoolCertificates.aspx. Accessed 14.12.20.
8. Kirkpatrick DL, Kirkpatrick JD. *Evaluating Training Programs: The Four Levels.* 3rd ed. San Francisco, CA: Berrett-Koehler Publishers; 2006.
9. Beck Dallaghan GL, Alerte AM, Ryan MS, et al. Enlisting community-based preceptor: a multi-center qualitative action study of U.S. pediatricians. *Acad Med.* 2017;92(8):1168–1174.
10. Christner JG, Beck Dallaghan GL, Briscoe G, et al. The community preceptor crisis: recruiting and retaining community-based faculty to teach medical students—a shared perspective from the Alliance for Clinical Education. *Teach Learn Med.* 2016;28(3):329–336.
11. Paul CR, Vercio C, Tenney Soeiro R, et al. The decline in community preceptor teaching activity: from the voices of pediatricians who have stopped teaching medical students. *Acad Med.* 2019. https://doi.org/10.1097/ACM.0000000000002947. ePub ahead of print.
12. Shaheen AW, Bossenbroek Fedoriw K, Khachaturyan S, et al. Aligning medical student curriculum with practice quality goals: impacts on quality metrics and practice capacity for students. *Am J Med.* 2019;132(12):1478–1483.
13. Goldman J, Kuper A, Wong BM. How theory can inform our understanding of experiential learning in quality improvement education. *Acad Med.* 2018;93(12):1784–1790.
14. Johnson Faherty L, Mate KS, Moses JM. Leveraging trainees to improve quality and safety at the point of care: three models for engagement. *Acad Med.* 2016;91(4):503–509.

7

Household-Centered Service-Learning: Florida International University Herbert Wertheim College of Medicine

Gregory W. Schneider, David R. Brown, and Luther Brewster

LEARNING OBJECTIVES

1. Describe the Florida International University Herbert Wertheim College of Medicine approach to household-centered service-learning, the Neighborhood Health Education Learning Program (NeighborhoodHELP).
2. Review the learning objectives and assessment strategies used in the Community-Engaged Physician courses that house NeighborhoodHELP.
3. Discuss the resources needed to implement and maintain NeighborhoodHELP.
4. Provide highlights from course evaluations and student and faculty perceptions of the program.
5. Offer advice for feasibility and sustainability of similar programs in different settings.

OUTLINE

CHAPTER SUMMARY

In this chapter, we describe the Neighborhood Health Education Learning Program and the accompanying Community-Engaged Physician courses at the Florida International University Herbert Wertheim College of Medicine. This longitudinal service-learning program, which launched in 2009, emphasizes ethics, social accountability, interprofessional teamwork, and the social determinants of health. Its focus is the delivery of care to the members of a household, with one person serving as the main point of contact. Care delivered at the household level enables student teams to play a distinctive and particularly valuable role within the health care system. Teams of medical, nursing, social work, and physician assistant students perform regular home visits in assigned underserved households throughout Miami-Dade County. During these visits, the students act as educators, coaches, navigators, and advocates, connecting household members to needed services and service providers. The program relies on a university-sponsored service support network of more than 20 outreach workers, three police officers, and partnerships with 7 colleges within the university, as well as more than 150 community service providers. Faculty assess students through a variety of mechanisms, from traditional quizzes and short-answer exams to reflection essays and point-of-care (workplace-based) assessments. From a curricular perspective, students experience the program under the umbrella of a series of courses, which they evaluate as well overall. Nevertheless, consistently identifying available time for students and households to meet remains a challenge. We close with suggestions for implementing similar programs elsewhere based on our successes and lessons learned.

INTRODUCTION

The Herbert Wertheim College of Medicine (HWCOM) at Florida International University (FIU) opened its doors to its first cohort of 43 medical students in the summer of 2009. This cohort was also the first to participate in the flagship program of the medical school, the Green Family Foundation Neighborhood Health Education Learning Program (NeighborhoodHELP). Since its inception, NeighborhoodHELP has been a longitudinal **service-learning** program in which students participate in home visits to assigned households as part of a broader, 4-year, interprofessional educational experience. The program allows students to take on a variety of **value-added roles**, with a focus on ethics, social accountability, interprofessional teamwork, and the **social determinants of health** (SDOH). The medical school gradually expanded until

2014, when it reached its target size of approximately 120 students per class cohort. As of 2019, HWCOM has graduated 612 students, all of whom participated in NeighborhoodHELP.

Context Within the HWCOM Curriculum

Designed to be a medical school that develops socially accountable, community-responsive physicians,[1] HWCOM does not have its own teaching hospital. Instead, it has formed partnerships with a number of local hospitals, health care systems, and providers. Throughout students' clinical experiences, from the early primary care and geriatrics preceptorships through the clerkships of their third and fourth years, they rotate at a variety of clinical locations across Miami-Dade County. This approach exposes students to a range of settings, patient populations, and practice models over the course of their training. Alongside their basic science, clinical medicine, and professional coursework and training, students engage in activities related to NeighborhoodHELP throughout the 4 years of medical school. The overarching curriculum for the school is organized into five strands: human biology; disease, illness, and injury; clinical medicine; professional development; and medicine and society. Within the medicine and society strand, students experience NeighborhoodHELP through a series of Community-Engaged Physician (CEP) courses. These courses focus on the core principles of health systems science, including interprofessional teamwork and the SDOH.

Conceptual Framework for the Program

In developing NeighborhoodHELP and the medicine and society strand, we relied on the organizing framework of community-oriented primary care (COPC) and service-oriented community-based education. As championed by Jack Geiger in the US, and based on the pioneering work of Sidney and Emily Kark in South Africa, COPC aims to be rooted in communities, for communities, and with communities.[2] Some of the key principles include targeting underserved populations, providing care without regard to ability to pay, looking at both individuals and communities as targets of intervention, involving community partners in program development and evaluation, and striving to address health disparities.[3,4] Recognizing that service-learning/community-based education takes a variety of forms, we aspired to develop a more robust approach that truly was based in, engaged with, and responsive to the needs of our local communities. Such a community-based approach would emphasize changing historical campus-community power dynamics, while simultaneously creating reciprocal partnerships between our medical school and the communities we serve.[5,6] Within the taxonomy delineated by Magzoub and Schmidt, NeighborhoodHELP is best described as *service-oriented community-based education* with concentrations on both health education and community development.[7]

The following sections outline the development and implementation of NeighborhoodHELP, with an emphasis on the value added to the households, to the local health system, and to our local communities. Next, these sections provide an overview of the concomitant CEP courses and the value added to the medical student experience. The chapter closes with a summary of the resources needed to initiate and sustain a similar program, recommendations for implementation, and reflections on successes and challenges.

DESCRIPTION OF NEIGHBORHOOD HEALTH EDUCATION LEARNING PROGRAM AT FLORIDA INTERNATIONAL UNIVERSITY HERBERT WERTHEIM COLLEGE OF MEDICINE

The core experience of NeighborhoodHELP involves teams of students and faculty performing home visits in vulnerable and medically underserved households in Miami-Dade County. These visits challenge students to address complex real-world medical, behavioral, social, environmental, ethical, and legal issues through a household-centered approach.[8] In exchange for helping to educate students, household members receive a variety of services, and the community at large receives numerous benefits that help to sustain household gains. We define "household" as a group of individuals residing together within a dwelling, and we define "household-centered care" as care that involves identifying and helping to manage the SDOH in ways that

can improve outcomes and quality of life for members of a household (Fig. 7.1).

Since we have more households, 850 as of June 2020, than the availability of approximately 360 student teams, we have households followed only by our outreach staff and households assigned to student teams. For those ~360 households assigned student teams, the core team includes medicine, nursing, social work, and/or physician assistant (PA) students; their supervising faculty; and community outreach workers. A typical team would include one faculty member, one medical student, one nursing student, one social work student, and one outreach worker. A medical student and nursing student work with one household. A social work student works with approximately 30 households.

A panel of faculty supervises household visits. As of September 2020, it includes 16 physician faculty employed by the medical school, two nursing faculty employed by the nursing school, and two PA faculty employed by the PA school. All faculty participate in a rotation. An appropriation from the state of Florida to medical schools funds the physician faculty and is part of HWCOM's core education budget. Household visits are considered an integral part of the teaching role of the core faculty. Grants and a philanthropic endowment fund other aspects of NeighborhoodHELP's community infrastructure and operations. This structure fosters financial sustainability and allows NeighborhoodHELP to stay in communities in perpetuity.

Prior to their fieldwork, medical students participate in a 5-month preparatory course, called Foundations for the Community-Engaged Physician, in their first year. This course and the full medicine and society strand of courses

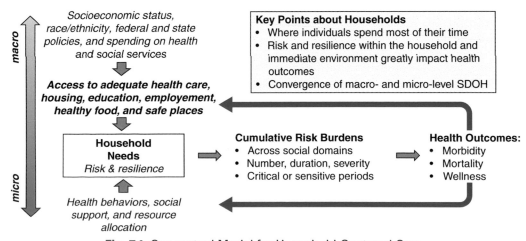

Fig. 7.1 Conceptual Model for Household-Centered Care.

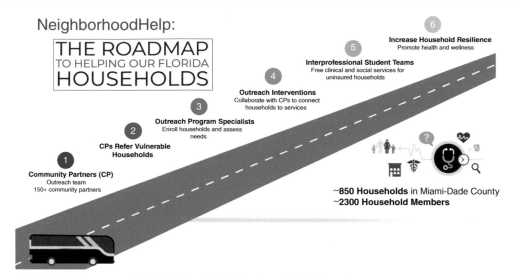

Fig. 7.2 The NeighborhoodHELP Roadmap.

are described later. During their fieldwork, teams assess, respond to, and longitudinally monitor SDOH. They identify risks and protective factors in their assigned households. More specifically, students—under faculty supervision—assess and research problems, connect household members to services in the community, and provide education and counseling. Depending on needs, the teams might engage professionals from other fields. For instance, when a team identifies an SDOH issue that is legally remediable, it will engage students and faculty from the law school's medical-legal partnership clinic. Similarly, if a household member would benefit from behavioral health services, master's-level social work students, working with behavioral health faculty and staff, provide counseling. Meanwhile, public health graduate students work on population health initiatives and education and premedical students provide tutoring, career advising, and educational counseling for both children and adults.[9] We envision these various student teams as one significant component of a larger integrated process in which we help to foster individual and household self-sufficiency (Fig. 7.2).

Laying the Groundwork for NeighborhoodHELP

Two years prior to dispatching the first student teams, faculty spent significant time gauging two key areas of community readiness: (1) the potential to amplify diverse community perspectives; and (2) community perception of the university. This informal process was informed by the foundations of community-campus partnerships for health[10] and community-based participatory research.[11]

Preparatory Work: Amplifying Diverse Community Perspectives

The goal was to introduce a disruptive approach to community partnership development that included more community stakeholders and, therefore, more perspectives in the discussion of what a medical school should do for its community. To facilitate this inclusion, we pledged (1) to expand our network beyond well-established community representatives and (2) to decline representation on community boards, committees, and task forces. Universities are consolidators of power. When they partner with established community organizations, they can inadvertently produce a gatekeeper relationship between the established community organization and the community.[12] Furthermore, this traditional method of partnership locks out alternative perspectives and can even reinforce a sense of hopelessness throughout the community. By collaborating with organizations and stakeholders typically overlooked or crowded out of discussions, we amplified their voices and thereby diversified the perspectives being discussed in the community.

Preparatory Work: Community Perception of the University

The initial stages of assessing readiness involved multiple formal and informal meetings with community stakeholders. Various organizational representatives attended these meetings. We began the process by opening a dialogue with the groups that had been most vocal in their disagreement with some of the university's prior community efforts. The approach offered an ability to address the long-standing concerns of these groups and helped distinguish NeighborhoodHELP from previous interfaces between the institution and the community.

Next, the NeighborhoodHELP leadership team conducted a door-to-door survey of 1845 households in the target neighborhoods to assess community needs and strengths.[13] This survey underscored a critical need for enhanced primary and preventive care services in these communities. To address this need, we ultimately opened a fleet of mobile health centers (MHCs), purchased by the medical school, which offer a range of integrated primary care, behavioral, and preventive services. Over time, the clinical leadership team for the MHCs set up collaborations with dental, radiology, and specialty providers in the area to provide access to care for members of participating households.

The Outreach Team

To ensure continuity of relationships with our community partners and households, we created a community outreach team. These outreach staff members support the students, recruit households, facilitate communication between households and student teams, and broker services through an extended network of community partners. We organized the outreach team into tiers that enable targeted work at the household, organizational, and policy levels. The program managers provide services and maintain relationships with community agencies that, in turn, refer households to the program. This arrangement fosters reciprocity, with partners providing referrals of households and with the households and communities benefiting from NeighborhoodHELP services. We strive to recruit and hire program specialists from the communities being served. These outreach specialists visit referred households to enroll them in the program, assess and address needs, and provide support to assigned student teams. While present in the neighborhoods where teams are operating, designated FIU police officers monitor the safety of teams and communicate with students, other team members, and local police. During separate and independent visits, the officers provide gun safety training and supply gunlocks to household members with firearms. Finally, policy coordinators create and oversee targeted programs aimed at promoting policies and services that facilitate healthy lifestyles. Along with the entire outreach team, they help communities become empowered, healthy, and resilient.

Scheduling household visits requires a significant amount of coordination. Students consult with their households to schedule visits, and a scheduling office assigns faculty to supervise the students. A proprietary case management digital platform—the NeighborhoodHELP Portal—facilitates household enrollment and maintenance, online visit scheduling, outcome tracking, and interdisciplinary communication. Once a household agrees to participate, an outreach program specialist visits the household, enrolls all interested members of the household, and does an initial assessment of the SDOH. Once a household agrees to student home visits, the initial visits focus on developing rapport and assessing needs. Gradually, the student team develops a holistic care plan to address social and medical needs and, as indicated, provides direct services (e.g., offering health education and/or counseling, facilitating food stamp applications, addressing immigration issues) via home visits and asynchronous work. As needed, the student teams also refer households to services, such as job training, food banks, and rental assistance, provided by our network of partners and to our MHCs for primary care. Faculty and student teams provide, on average, three household visits per year. The visits last approximately 1 hour, plus additional 30-minute "huddles" by the team before and after each visit. Students communicate monthly with their households to follow up on household needs and care plans and to coordinate visits and services with team members. Students document status and interactions in the portal and electronic health record (EHR) to track household progress over time. The process of assessment and service provision occurs iteratively throughout the program. Students periodically assess and reflect on their efforts. Prior to graduation, students work with their assigned household to develop a plan for transitioning it either out of the program or to a new student team.

Using the categories of **value-added roles** articulated by Jed Gonzalo and his team at Penn State College of Medicine,[14] we feel that NeighborhoodHELP adds value to the patients, households, and communities we serve in a number of ways. On the patient level, our student teams provide patient education, facilitate patient access to services and resources, and assist in monitoring patient progress in accordance with care plans. They also facilitate partnerships with households via coaching and health promotion and provide psychological and emotional support for household members. On the clinical level, the student teams facilitate communication among medical and behavioral health providers and coordination with local social service providers. The teams whose households take advantage of the MHC assist our primary care physicians in gathering more comprehensive patient assessments. All student teams are tasked with assisting in referral follow-up, and some students take on additional quality improvement tasks, aimed to improve our MHC clinical operations and processes. These clinical **value-added roles**, in turn, add value to the local health system by fostering better care coordination and by decreasing inappropriate emergency department and hospital utilization.

LEARNING GOALS

All medical students are required to participate in NeighborhoodHELP through their CEP courses, which fall within the medicine and society strand of the medical school. The community-based education structure of these courses places the SDOH at the core of the curriculum, provides students with a rich longitudinal clinical experience, and reinforces our interprofessional, household-centered approach to health care.

Within the taxonomy of service learning by Magzoub and colleagues, service-oriented community-based education involves programs that engage their students and staff in actual service delivery. Traditionally, almost all of the programs found in this category are in less economically developed countries, but we find the approach works just as well in vulnerable and underserved communities in the US. Internationally, the services provided range from primary care and preventive services to broader community development and mobilization.[7] NeighborhoodHELP consciously embraces a wide range of health and development services and, like the international examples, began its work with an assessment of needs and resources in the targeted communities.

Striving to improve the health of those communities and of household members, students apply the ethical, social, behavioral, and clinical knowledge and skills they learn throughout their curriculum. To guide that curriculum, we outlined social accountability competencies that HWCOM medical students aim to master by graduation (Table 7.1).

Through NeighborhoodHELP and their CEP courses, students have the opportunity to develop and apply these competencies through real-world activities designed to improve health and well-being. Although the emphasis is social accountability and the **social determinants of health**, many of these competencies also involve the knowledge, skills, and attitudes involved in the other domains of health systems science.

The Medicine and Society Strand and Curricular and Co-Curricular Integration

As mentioned earlier, each HWCOM course is set within one of five longitudinal curriculum strands—(1) human biology; (2) disease, illness, and injury; (3) clinical medicine; (4) professional development; and (5) medicine and society. All strands run concurrently across four sequential "periods" of study, with each period loosely following an academic year. While maximizing horizontal and vertical

TABLE 7.1 **Herbert Wertheim College of Medicine Social Accountability Competency Domain and Critical Competencies**
SOCIAL ACCOUNTABILITY (SA): Working collaboratively to meet the health needs of patients and society to demonstrate improved health outcomes and reduce health disparities.
SA 1.   Demonstrate an understanding of the influence and potential implications of social determinants of health on beliefs, behaviors, and outcomes, and incorporate this knowledge into patient care.
SA 2.   Identify and utilize appropriate sources of information to analyze significant public health issues, applying data to reach defensible conclusions.
SA 3.   Accurately describe the organization and basic financial models of the US health care system and potential impact of this system on patients for whom the student has provided care.
SA 4.   Accept and report personal biases and errors, identify potential sources of errors, and develop action plans to reduce risk of future errors.
SA 5.   Collaborate with stakeholders inside and outside the health care system to coordinate optimal care and improve health.
SA 6.   Apply knowledge of health advocacy, systems, and policy to identify strategies for reducing health disparities and promoting individual and population health.

integration, the strands help organize all educational objectives and courses within the school of medicine. The medicine and society strand focuses on the social sciences and the impact of **social determinants of health** and health care. Each medicine and society strand course has one or two course directors who oversee the educational enterprises for the course (Fig. 7.3). In period 1, prior to their first household visit, students take two courses in the strand: Ethical Foundations of Medicine and Foundations for the Community-Engaged Physician. Through these courses, students participate in didactic and small group learning sessions that focus on ethics, the socioeconomic and cultural aspects of health, community engagement, interprofessional teamwork, patient-centered communication, and motivational interviewing. In period 2, under the umbrella of CEP I, students begin their household visits. Alongside the four required visits that academic year, they

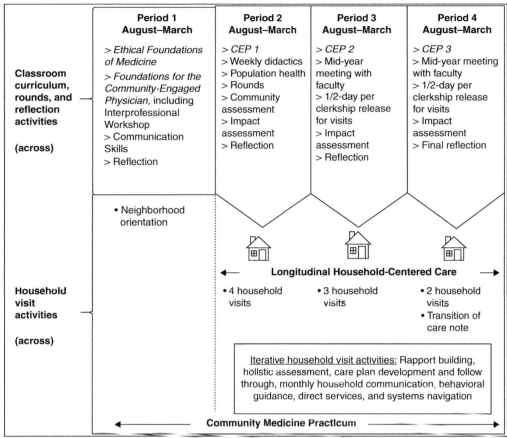

Fig. 7.3 The Medicine and Society Curriculum Strand. NeighborhoodHELP classroom activities align with service to households and community partners, periodic reflection, and the assessment of impact. This figure reflects the longitudinal coordination of classroom learning, rounds, and reflection activities (*top row*) with student household visit activities (*bottom row*). These intertwined classroom and household visit activities unfold across the four periods (loosely aligned with traditional academic years) of the medical school curriculum (*columns*). Student household visits, represented by the house, begin in period 2, and initially focus on assessing health needs in the context of SDOH and on developing a holistic plan to address identified needs. Subsequently, student teams provide direct services—such as health education, health coaching, and care coordination—to household members.

have ongoing didactic and experiential learning activities that align with the *Healthy People 2020* leading health indicators and social determinants.[15] The course contains other content—including policy, medical-legal partnerships, preventive medicine, and behavioral health—to help build the knowledge, skills, and attitudes needed for meaningful interactions with household and community members. In periods 3 and 4, during the clerkship and senior clinical periods, classroom activities are curtailed. To accomplish three visits in period 3 and two in period 4, the students

receive release time during their clerkships and rotations. While these courses are positioned within the medicine and society strand, their core principles—ethics and the SDOH—are integrated into preclinical cases and clinical activities across the 4-year curriculum. In addition, we integrate content from other strands, in particular, clinical medicine and professional development, into various activities within NeighborhoodHELP. For example, communication skills—integral to the services that students provide through their household visits—are presented as part of the students' clinical skills course. Meanwhile, structured household health education activities reinforce relevant basic and clinical science subjects.

One final layer of co-curricular integration involves integration of the community medicine practicum with the HWCOM Panther Learning Communities (PLCs), an educational and social structure that promotes a sense of community within the school. We divide the entire student body and core faculty among four PLCs. Each PLC aligns itself with geographic areas served by NeighborhoodHELP. Student leaders within each PLC oversee programs in NeighborhoodHELP target areas that address identified community needs (e.g., education pipeline activities, health education, screening services, support for women's health services, and health system policy initiatives). By training and empowering medical students to create and administer programs, the PLCs complement and support the medicine and society strand curriculum. These student-run programs are supported by staff from our Office of Student Affairs and offer additional resources to NeighborhoodHELP households, community partners, and student teams. Some PLC activities are entirely extracurricular, while time spent in "practicum-approved" activities counts toward a 30-hour practicum requirement. Activities are reviewed by a committee including student affairs staff, medicine and society faculty, and NeighborhoodHELP outreach staff. To be approved for practicum credit, activities must have appropriate oversight, target population health competencies, and provide benefit to NeighborhoodHELP neighborhoods, households, or partner organizations. The integration of the PLCs with NeighborhoodHELP brings the institution, students, and faculty into an extended network that engages collaboratively with the communities that HWCOM is committed to serving.

We contend that the community-focused approach of NeighborhoodHELP, of the medicine and society strand courses, and of the PLCs provide students with a value-added medical education in a number of ways. Within the professional development framework for **value-added roles** laid out by Gonzalo and colleagues, a value-added education provides enriching "opportunities for students to learn not only biomedicine but also how biomedicine plays out in real-world health systems."[16] NeighborhoodHELP offers such opportunities throughout its operations. Students, for instance, learn to work with interprofessional partners both in classroom exercises and in real-world scenarios with their households. By functioning as health coaches and health educators in the household, students hone their clinical skills, while also learning to better appreciate the patient experience, gaining insight into the perspective of another while seated in their homes. While acting as navigators and trying to identify community resources, medical students become better attuned to the complicated structure of health care and social services in the US. Doing so alongside social work and nursing students and faculty challenges medical students to see those structures from the perspectives of different disciplines. The monthly phone calls to households, the emails and portal postings to interprofessional colleagues, and the in-home clinical encounters provide students with the chance to enhance their communication skills in ways they typically would not be able to until they were on clinical rotations. In the manner that Gonzalo and colleagues have described as educating "systems aware physicians," NeighborhoodHELP challenges our students to think of themselves as part of a complex system and as members of a team striving to provide patient-centered care.[17]

TECHNIQUES TO ASSESS LEARNERS

Given the multidimensional nature of NeighborhoodHELP and of the CEP courses, we have taken a multimodal approach to student assessment. Our overarching methodology aligns with the work of Miller and colleagues on assessment in higher education, with their emphasis on assessment that is both pragmatic and informed by research. As they contend, we see the principal functions of assessment as being threefold: (1) to provide systematic indications of the quality of students' learning for both students and instructors, (2) to ensure the maintenance of standards in professional education, and (3) to motivate students throughout the course of their studies. In addition, we strive to vary the assessments and match them to the particular learning format and educational objectives of a particular session or unit.[18] As an outgrowth of our participation in the Association of American Medical Colleges Core EPA pilot,[19] we developed direct observation activity-focused assessment tools that could be used when faculty were in the field doing home visits[20] and could provide formative feedback to students, while being adaptable to a variety of settings.[21] The assessments needed to be housed in particular courses. Thus, we mapped out the assignments and assessments across the courses to ensure both continuity and reinforcement, while reducing redundancy. All courses in the entire medicine and society strand are pass/fail. Our approach to assessment in each of the four courses that comprise the CEP series is described next.

Foundations for the Community-Engaged Physician—Period 1

In period 1, the Foundations for the CEP course runs 16 weeks over a 5-month period in the fall and winter. The course introduces students to the SDOH, health disparities, health equity, and interprofessional teamwork. Sessions focus on a range of topics, from particular determinants, such as food or housing insecurity to the disparities faced by different socioeconomic, racial, and ethnic groups. The emphasis is on elucidating problems, and then providing practical solutions for physicians of various disciplines. All didactic sessions are 2 hours, with most sessions having a similar format, in which a small group activity follows an introductory lecture. The final three sessions are more practical, with a live role-play of how a household visit unfolds, an introduction to the EHR used on household visits, and a large interprofessional workshop. The workshop is the largest educational event the medical school hosts each year, involving ~450 students from nine different disciplines within three different colleges in the university.

The assessments in this course take the following forms: brief quizzes, small-group activity worksheets, a short-answer midterm, a small-group reflection paper, and an individual reflection paper. For approximately half of the class sessions, students will have a preclass reading from our course textbook, *Medical Management of Vulnerable and Underserved Patients: Principles, Practice, and Populations, 2nd edition,* and a quiz on that reading during the session. The lecture reinforces and augments the reading. Throughout the course, the cohort of ~120 students is broken into in-class activity groups of about six students. During the active learning portions of class, the groups collaboratively complete a task-oriented worksheet related to the SDOH and addressing health disparities that they turn in together. For the interprofessional workshop, all students watch brief modules instructing the future physicians about the work of other disciplines. Faculty from the different disciplines compile the modules, and our students take a brief quiz after each module. Midway through the course, students have a take-home short essay midterm on the SDOH and health disparities. At the end of the course, students write a brief reflection paper and participate in a group reflection on a film. The course is organized around the theme of justice; all small groups watch a film, chosen by them, that touches on that theme. Students individually and collectively reflect on the film and what it taught them about fairness and justice.

Community-Engaged Physician I—Period 2

The second year of medical school launches the full NeighborhoodHELP experience with CEP I. The course includes 24 weeks of didactic sessions and 4 interprofessional household visits, spread over a full year. About one-half of the didactic sessions follow the format initiated in Foundations for the CEP, in which an introductory lecture leads into an in-class small group activity. These sessions cover topics such as chronic disease management, ethical

challenges faced doing home visits, preventive medicine guidelines and counseling, and health systems science topics, such as strategies for handoffs that foster patient safety. The remaining sessions take on a variety of formats, including traditional lectures, "meet the patient" sessions, a built environment design thinking workshop, reflection rounds, and interprofessional rounds. Reflections rounds involve faculty facilitating small groups of medical students from the same PLC discussing their experiences in NeighborhoodHELP in response to a handful of prompts and guiding questions. Interprofessional rounds involve PLC-specific teams of medical, nursing, and social work students presenting their households, discussing the issues faced by their households, and brainstorming potential solutions together.

The household visits occur quarterly. Teams of medical and nursing students, sometimes along with a social work student, coordinate with their assigned supervising faculty member to plan, proceed with, and debrief the visit. As part of their course requirements, medical students complete at least one household activity during each visit. A household activity is a structured health education, information gathering, or health/lifestyle counseling intervention designed by our core faculty for medical students to pursue in conjunction with their interprofessional partners. There are now 13 options available for students to choose; examples include nutritional guidance, a home safety assessment, a collaborative behavioral guidance activity based on motivational interviewing, and a childhood asthma coaching protocol. In CEP I, students must complete an SDOH assessment activity and a preventive medicine counseling activity sometime during the course of the year.

The assessments tied to the range of didactic activities in CEP I include the following: brief quizzes, small-group activity worksheets, a short-answer midterm, an individual reflection paper, rounds rubrics, and a group community medicine research paper. For the household visits, we have designed a global workplace-based assessment (WBA) for the visit and shorter WBAs tied to each structured household activity. The multiple-choice quizzes, small-group worksheets, and short-answer midterm function similarly as in the period 1 course. The individual reflection paper in CEP I links with reflection rounds and involves the same guiding prompt: "What has working with your household taught you about the SDOH?" The paper rubric focuses on the depth of the thought and reflection and on the quality of the writing. The three interprofessional rounds and the one reflection round all have accompanying rubrics completed by the facilitating faculty. The rubrics assess domains related to professionalism, presentation skills, and group processing skills, along with HSS skills, such as working with teammates and engagement with household needs and the SDOH. The community medicine research paper is a group project, involving around six students from the same PLC, with a focus on a health disparity noted in one of their NeighborhoodHELP communities. The groups write a formal public health proposal. Faculty grade the paper according to a structured rubric assessing their literature search, their appraisal of the community and cultural context, and the strength of their proposed intervention. The WBAs tied to household visits are short, electronic Qualtrics rubrics that faculty complete within 48 hours of the visit. The student receives a copy by email. The rubrics assess domains that we have labelled "functions," including things such as team communications, quality of preparation and follow-up, acknowledgment of limitations, patient-centeredness, and attentiveness to the SDOH. To ensure that students are maintaining an ongoing relationship with their households, we also perform monthly audits of the portal documentation to see that students have recorded their monthly communication with their households and interprofessional partners.

Community-Engaged Physician II and III— Periods 3 and 4

In the final two years of medical school, students continue with the home visit experiences of NeighborhoodHELP, while no longer having didactic sessions. The format for these visits remains unchanged and, in the ideal, students continue with their same assigned households over 3 years. If students are having difficulty scheduling appointments with their households—say, due to a job change for a household member or because a household has withdrawn from the program or moved—they are reassigned. Students have three household visits in their third year, under the aegis of CEP II, and two in the final year in the CEP III course. In addition to their household visits, fourth-year students have a half-hour mentoring session with a matched first-year student, who is about to start CEP I, to provide advice and guidance on NeighborhoodHELP, according to a structured mentoring worksheet. We have designed both CEP II and III to provide brief midpoint opportunities for students to meet with an assigned faculty NeighborhoodHELP mentor, give a formal presentation about one of their household members, and discuss any next steps.

The assessments in these periods 3 and 4 courses match the endeavors described. After the household visits, students receive feedback via WBAs on the visits themselves and on any household activities pursued. At the midpoint of the academic year, students arrange for a meeting with their assigned NeighborhoodHELP faculty mentor. During the meeting, the students give a formal oral presentation, similar to a clinical history and physical, which is graded according to a checklist rubric. At the conclusion of both

courses, students write individual reflection papers on their service-learning experiences of the prior year. The prompts for the papers change, with the students challenged to think more about their professional identity and development. Third-year students are asked to reflect on the question: "How has working with your household affected the way you interact with patients in general?" Fourth-year students receive the prompt: "As medical school comes to a close, how has working with your household(s) affected how you think of yourself as a future physician?" The paper rubrics assess the quality of the writing and the depth of thought and reflection. For their end-of-year mentoring session with a soon-to-be second-year student, the fourth-year students complete a mentoring worksheet that they upload to their Canvas Learning Management Platform. In accordance with the three principle functions of assessment outlined at the outset of this section, we are continually adjusting some of the rubrics and the timing of different assessment activities. Our guiding approach remains threefold: providing systematic indications of the quality of student work, ensuring competency standards throughout all of our courses, and striving to keep students engaged and motivated.

EVALUATION PROCEDURES

All courses at HWCOM undergo a formal evaluation process coordinated by the Office of Medical Education (OME). At the conclusion of each course, students receive an electronic questionnaire that they are required to complete. The questionnaire includes five Likert scale questions and the opportunity for free text comments. After the questionnaire results are tabulated and compiled, the OME provides them with the course directors and arranges for a 1-hour course debriefing with our curriculum deans and with student representatives who provide additional feedback on the course.

The standard Likert scale questions, with a low-to-high scoring range from 1 to 5, are the following: (1) The course content (lectures, materials, activities) matched the learning objectives; (2) The assignment or activities were relevant and supported the course content; (3) The course was well organized; (4) The course director communicated effectively with students and faculty; and (5) This course fostered my learning. Having standard questions allows for comparison across courses and over time. The free text comments and course de-briefing sessions allow for more qualitative feedback, which can be considered during annual revisions to the course content and design.

Over the history of the CEP courses, students have gradually evaluated the courses higher and higher by Likert-scale tabulations and have offered more frequent positive narrative comments. Students tend to rate the first-year course the highest in the series, citing the overall design of the course, the passion of the instructors, and the creativity of the small-group learning activities. Many students comment on NeighborhoodHELP as being eye opening and one of the main reasons that they chose FIU over other schools. Seeing the college's mission to be community focused and to create socially accountable physicians through these courses is also heartening for the students. Fourth-year students frequently comment on how NeighborhoodHELP was valuable for them on the residency interview trail, as it gave them experiences and insights that helped them stand out from other students.

Given the complicated structure of NeighborhoodHELP and the CEP courses, students have expressed general frustration about the communication regarding course assignments and, in particular, regarding the difficulties scheduling household visits. To improve communication, the course directors have created "student engagement checklists" for all four CEP courses, with a one-page listing of all course assignments and due dates. For CEP I, II, and III, the course directors also send out course-specific monthly newsletters, reminding students of any assignments due that month and offering tips for completing those assignments. Improving the household visit scheduling process has been a longer-term project—we have initiated a number of mechanisms to facilitate easier scheduling. The most important improvement was the launch of an online visit scheduler in 2018, in which students could reserve a spot on an electronic calendar integrated into a portal and overseen by our scheduling office. The platform continually updates, allowing students to see when the program has available faculty and safety officer coverage, so that they can negotiate appointment times with their teammates and households live. The online scheduler has been one of the crucial ways in which we have improved the workflow for our students, and it shows up frequently on our course evaluations.

IMPLEMENTATION HISTORY AND STRATEGIES EMPLOYED

While envisioning NeighborhoodHELP and the curricular apparatus to support the student experience of the program, we proceeded along the lines of the Kern model for curricular development, also mentioned in Part 3 of this book.[22] In the model, step five focuses on implementation. According to this framework, the crucial aspects of implementation are (1) obtain political support, (2) secure resources, (3) address barriers, (4) introduce the curriculum, and (5) administer the curriculum. In describing these steps, we will also highlight resources needed and key advice for feasibility and sustainability.

Kern Implementation Step 1: Obtain Political Support

The idea of community-based education preceded the opening of the medical school itself and was always a vital part of the mission and community focus of HWCOM. The current mission statement of the college explicitly mentions preparing "socially accountable, community-based physicians, scientists, and health professionals"—in-home experiences have been considered integral to accomplishing these mission goals. The founding dean, John Rock, and the founding chair of the Department of Humanities, Health, and Society at HWCOM, Pedro Greer, Jr., championed the idea of NeighborhoodHELP and garnered support for the project in all of his initial hires for the college of medicine. Prior to signing any clinical staff, they enlisted the help of a team of social scientists, who guided the initial program development. The early faculty and staff then consulted with community stakeholders, including the local county hospital system, the county public health department, other county officials, larger community-based organizations such as the Greater Miami Jewish Federation, and a variety of small grassroots organizations. Providing technical support to local organizations, and providing direct services to their clients, served (and serves) as an ongoing source of community-based social capital. The social science team conducted a needs assessment in targeted communities identified by these initial partners and stakeholders; that needs assessment, along with consultations with these founding stakeholders, laid the groundwork for a variety of further community partnerships. When the strand structure for the curriculum began to take shape, Dr. Rock and Dr. Greer fought for the establishment of the medicine and society strand to be the curricular home for the social accountability features of HWCOM. By incorporating the courses that support NeighborhoodHELP into the strand structure of the college of medicine, the program has become central to the educational efforts of the school.

RESOURCES NEEDED

Kern Implementation Step 2: Secure Resources

Knowing that a complex health and social service delivery platform outside the context of a hospital or a community health center would require a constellation of support in terms of money, personnel, and community partners, the founding faculty worked to establish an endowment for the program. Initially funded by local philanthropists, the Green Family Foundation and the Batchelor Foundation, they secured a stable source of revenue for the program. Some of the very first support staff hired included the outreach team in order to have a core workforce that would initiate and sustain relationships with community partners and households. The outreach specialists, in particular, were, and are, hired from the communities we serve. The community partners, in addition to serving as a source of household referrals, provide a resource network for students and outreach members to obtain needed services for households. This approach provides connections to those communities and a unique perspective that shapes how the whole program interacts with community service providers and clients. Finally, Dean Rock committed core educational funding for core NeighborhoodHELP clinician faculty who would specifically be tasked with overseeing household visits weekly.

KEY ADVICE FOR FEASIBILITY AND SUSTAINABILITY

Kern Implementation Step 3: Address Barriers

Securing such lines of funding also took into account one anticipated barrier: the concern that part-time faculty would not prioritize the household-centered educational experience. One of the ways in which this barrier was addressed included committing the core faculty to full-time teaching without clinically based incentives to distract from core educational roles. NeighborhoodHELP faculty, for instance, teach weekly in clinical skills courses, in problem-based learning sessions for third-year students, and in case-based learning sessions for first- and second-year students in basic science courses. Establishing a program like NeighborhoodHELP has the potential to alienate faculty and departments involved in functions more clearly aligned with traditional medical education, such as basic science educators, core clinical departments, and offices to support student performance on the boards and in doing well in the match. Our approach to this potential challenge has been to partner with those departments and offices, collaborating on joint curricular initiatives and helping them achieve their goals, while offering complementary experiences in our courses. The community network has facilitated SDOH-focused service referrals, enabling the student teams to address barriers to health in their assigned households.

Kern Implementation Step 4: Introduce the Curriculum and Kern Step 5: Administer the Curriculum

The medicine and society strand courses launched as part of the initial curriculum at HWCOM. The design, learning activities, and assessment strategies involved in the initial courses have changed significantly over time, but what has sustained and improved them has been the flexible oversight structure we have in place. For the CEP I, II, and III courses, in particular, we have established a course administrators' committee that advises the two course directors on all aspects of the didactic portions. For administrative support, these three courses have two full-time administrative assistants who help with the course in both its didactic and household visit aspects. With all of the difficulties in overseeing a program that provides about 1200 home visits yearly, the two course directors meet weekly with their administrative support staff to review student emails and offer solutions to any problems. In addition, this oversight team has a weekly phone meeting with one of the outreach directors to discuss specific households that have presented particularly difficult challenges for our students. Finally, the CEP course directors host a yearly half-day retreat for all core NeighborhoodHELP faculty and outreach workers, plus interprofessional faculty and medical student representatives, where we review all operations of NeighborhoodHELP in order to celebrate successes and look for opportunities for improvement.

CONCLUSION

This dedication to ongoing monitoring, to gathering feedback from stakeholders, and to striving for improvement characterizes the FIU approach to value-added medical education. Within this approach, NeighborhoodHELP and the CEP courses act as complementary pillars that support the broader mission of HWCOM to foster socially accountable, community-responsive physicians. Built on a network of community partners supported by the work of our outreach team, NeighborhoodHELP offers value to households and health care systems in the communities served. Through their home visits, interprofessional student teams support the work of local primary care clinicians and connect households to local social service providers and resources. These household-centered care efforts can help participants address the SDOH, build resilience, and ultimately achieve better health outcomes.

To initiate and implement NeighborhoodHELP and its supporting curricula, the founding deans and faculty took proactive steps to ensure that the program had secure endowment funding and a core set of faculty dedicated to the enterprise. To facilitate collaboration with other departments and operations within the medical school, those faculty teach across many courses within the school. Recognizing the complex nature of the enterprise, we have put in place a number of ways to monitor various aspects of the program, from multidimensional student assessments to regular course evaluations, from weekly team meetings to yearly retreats. We continue to strive for improving communication with our students and among various stakeholders within the program and to make for easier scheduling of household visits. In collaboration with our outreach team, we aspire to keep evolving in ways that benefit the experiences of our students and our households.

STUDENT REFLECTIONS

Foundations for the Community-Engaged Physician

"This course is a must for all future physicians."

"The course had really concise lectures which taught so much important information and really helped me grasp a true understanding of the different factors that play a role in the access to and delivery of health care. The professors are some of the most passionate individuals I have ever met, and this course was very valuable."

"Overall I thoroughly enjoyed this course. I think the course is organized very well and brings up many important parts of medicine that don't get covered in other courses or during other aspects of medical training. This course really sets FIU apart from other medical schools and really gets to the heart of our school's mission."

"I greatly appreciate the course, and its mission is the reason I chose FIU as a medical school. As Virchow said, 'The physicians are the natural attorneys of the poor, and the social problems should largely be solved by them.' I appreciate this course because it helps to instill this lesson."

Community-Engaged Physician I, II, and III

"This class allowed us the opportunity to absorb so many different kinds of information regarding social determinants of health … I truly enjoyed all the information learned from this class."

"I thought the course was well taught and organized considering the unpredictability of [NeighborhoodHELP] [and our households]."

"I enjoyed working with my [household] in the [NeighborhoodHELP] program and continuing care with the patients in my [household]. Faculty are all excellent and worked with me very well during the site visits. CEP program was also very reasonable in helping me schedule visits. Thank you!"

"This is a great course. It allows us to refine our clinical and communication skills in the field. I really enjoy working with my household."

REFERENCES

1. Oandasan I, Malik R, Waters I, Lambert-Lanning A. Being community-responsive physicians. Doing the right thing. *Can Fam Physician*. 2004;50:1004–1010.
2. Geiger HJ. Community-oriented primary care: the legacy of Sidney Kark. *Am J Public Health*. 1993;83(7):946–947. https://doi.org/10.2105/AJPH.83.7.946.
3. Geiger HJ. The first community health centers: a model of enduring value. *J Ambul Care Manag*. 2005;28(4):313–320. https://doi.org/10.1097/00004479-200510000-00006.
4. Geiger HJ. Community-oriented primary care: a path to community development. *Am J Public Health*. 2002;92(11):1713–1716. https://doi.org/10.2105/AJPH.92.11.1713.
5. CCPH Board of Directors. Position Statement on Authentic Partnerships. Published online 2013. https://ccphealth.org/95-2/principles-of-partnering/ Accessed December 15, 2020.
6. Hunt JB, Bonham C, Jones L. Understanding the goals of service learning and community-based medical education: a systematic review. *Acad Med*. 2011;86(2):246–251. https://doi.org/10.1097/ACM.0b013e3182046481.
7. Magzoub MEMA, Schmidt HG. A taxonomy of community-based medical education. *Acad Med*. 2000;75(7):699–707. https://doi.org/10.1097/00001888-200007000-00011.
8. Rock JA, Acuña JM, Lozano JM, et al. Impact of an academic–community partnership in medical education on community health: evaluation of a novel student-based home visitation program. *South Med J*. 2014;107(4):203–211. https://doi.org/10.1097/SMJ.0000000000000080.
9. Greer PJ, Brown DR, Brewster LG, et al. Socially accountable medical education: an innovative approach at Florida International University Herbert Wertheim College of Medicine. *Acad Med*. 2018;93(1):60–65. https://doi.org/10.1097/ACM.0000000000001811.
10. Bringle RG, Hatcher JA. Campus-community partnerships: the terms of engagement. *J Soc Issues*. 2002;58(3):503–516. https://doi.org/10.1111/1540-4560.00273.
11. Coombe CM, Schulz AJ, Guluma L, et al. Enhancing capacity of community–academic partnerships to achieve health equity: results from the CBPR Partnership Academy. *Health Promot Pract*. Published online December 29, 2018:152483991881883. https://doi.org/10.1177/1524839918818830.
12. Sandmann L, Kliewer B. Theoretical and applied perspectives on power: recognizing processes that undermine effective community-university partnerships. *J Community Engagem and Scholarsh*. 2012;5(2). http://jces.ua.edu/theoretical-and-applied-perspectives-on-power-recognizing-processes-that-undermine-effective-community-university-partnerships/. Published October 15, 2012. Accessed December 15, 2020.
13. Florida International University College of Medicine. Community benchmark executive summary Northwest Miami-Dade. Published online 2010. http://digitalcommons.fiu.edu/com_archival/709. Accessed December 15, 2020.
14. Gonzalo JD, Dekhtyar M, Hawkins RE, Wolpaw DR. How can medical students add value? Identifying roles, barriers,

and strategies to advance the value of undergraduate medical education to patient care and the health system. *Acad Med.* 2017;92(9):1294–1301. https://doi.org/10.1097/ACM.0000000000001662.

15. Institute of Medicine (US) Committee on Leading Health Indicators for *Healthy People 2020*. Leading health indicators for *Healthy People 2020*: Letter Report. National Academies Press (US); 2011. http://www.ncbi.nlm.nih.gov/books/NBK209475/. Accessed December 15, 2020.

16. Gonzalo JD, Thompson BM, Haidet P, Mann K, Wolpaw DR. A constructive reframing of student roles and systems learning in medical education using a communities of practice lens. *Acad Med.* 2017;92(12):1687–1694. https://doi.org/10.1097/ACM.0000000000001778.

17. Gonzalo JD, Wolpaw D, Graaf D, Thompson BM. Educating patient-centered, systems-aware physicians: a qualitative analysis of medical student perceptions of value-added clinical systems learning roles. *BMC Med Educ.* 2018;18(1). https://doi.org/10.1186/s12909-018-1345-5.

18. Miller AH, Imrie BW, Cox K. *Student Assessment in Higher Education: A Handbook for Assessing Performance.* London: Kogan Page; 1998.

19. Obeso V, Brown D, Aiyer M, et al. *Core Entrustable Professional Activities for Entering Residency: Toolkits for the 13 Core EPAs.* Washington, DC: Association of American Medical Colleges; 2017.

20. Bryan C, Clegg K, eds. *Innovative Assessment in Higher Education.* London: Routledge; 2006.

21. Gibbs G, Simpson C. Measuring the response of students to assessment: the Assessment Experience Questionnaire. In: *11th International Improving Student Learning Symposium, Hinkley. Semantic Scholar.* Published online 2003. https://www.semanticscholar.org/paper/Measuring-the-response-of-students-to-assessment%3A-Gibbs-Simpson/57111701f9d713bde7780f6442e6bb4c1cf1b43b. Accessed May 12, 2021.

22. Kern DE, Thomas PA, Hughes MT, eds. *Curriculum Development for Medical Education: A Six-Step Approach.* 2nd ed. Baltimore, MD: Johns Hopkins University Press; 2009.

8

Early Medical Students as Clinical Microsystem Agents of Change— Improving Quality, Value, and the Patient Experience: University of California, San Francisco, School of Medicine

Stephanie Rennke, Leslie Sheu, and Anna Chang

LEARNING OBJECTIVES

1. Define the theoretical context for early medical students serving as health systems agents of change to improve quality, value, equity, and the patient experience.
2. Describe the goals and curriculum for a preclerkship experiential health systems improvement curriculum.
3. Compare and contrast four sample student projects across clinical sites in the context of overall program outcome measures.
4. Articulate implementation resources, including faculty development and health system interprofessional teams.
5. Share best practices for feasibility and sustainability for an education program that embeds early students in the clinical microsystem as value-added team members.

OUTLINE

CHAPTER SUMMARY

In this chapter, we highlight the University of California, San Francisco, School of Medicine Clinical Microsystem Clerkship (CMC) as an example of a curriculum that embeds preclerkship students in the microsystem as team members and agents of change. We review the CMC curriculum as well as the roles and responsibilities of the students, faculty coaches, and the interprofessional team. Finally, we discuss this program's 5-year implementation outcomes, lessons learned, and best practices.

INTRODUCTION

Physicians in the 21st century are challenged with the responsibility of improving quality and value in care delivery within complex health systems. To address these challenges, medical schools are beginning to add expectations of competence in **health systems science** (HSS) in order to graduate physicians capable of not only thriving as clinicians, educators, or researchers but also as leaders and partners in health systems improvement.[1-3] While there are multiple models for incorporating HSS into undergraduate medical education, there is growing interest in embedding medical students into longitudinal value-added roles in the clinical workplace. These efforts can provide direct involvement in HSS activities that have an impact on clinical care and improve quality, patient safety, value, access to care, and health care disparities.[4] This chapter describes a curriculum that enables medical students to serve as contributing team members of health care systems to add value by completing a project that improves an important process or outcome to benefit patients, physicians, other health care professionals, or the system.

To introduce medical students to HSS, we have employed two theoretical lenses to guide our strategy: (1) **communities of practice** and (2) **workplace learning**. Communities of practice learning theory, described by Lave and Wenger in 1991, asserts that people working in the same environment learn together within its social construct.[5] Thus, communities of practice "are groups of people who share a concern or a passion for something they do and learn how to do it better as they interact regularly."[4] Through intentional interactions, the group works collaboratively toward a shared purpose by building knowledge and relationships.[6] Similarly, workplace learning and experiential learning are concepts based on sociocultural theory that learning occurs "on the job," through attainment of new knowledge and skills in both formal and informal ways.[7,8] Traditionally, early medical students learned in classrooms or in limited shadowing clinical experiences. Through experiential engagement in HSS, medical students can be integrated into clinical communities of practice with value-added roles to gain insight into the culture and dynamics of the clinical workplace.

Educators have described barriers to implementing HSS into medical student education, including curricular time, resource investment, faculty development, student engagement, and learner assessment.[9] Despite the challenges, students can serve as agents of change when they are embedded into teams focused on current quality improvement projects.[10] Here, we describe the University of California, San Francisco (UCSF) Clinical Microsystem Clerkship (CMC), a longitudinal element in the school of medicine, in which early medical students bring value to clinical teams and contribute to real-time health care system improvements.

DESCRIPTION OF THE CLINICAL MICROSYSTEMS CLERKSHIP AT THE UNIVERSITY OF CALIFORNIA, SAN FRANCISCO, SCHOOL OF MEDICINE

Curriculum Overview

In 2016, the UCSF School of Medicine launched the Bridges curriculum, which revamped the entire school of medicine curriculum by incorporating foundational knowledge in basic and clinical sciences with HSS, allowing time for scientific discovery, providing dedicated time for scholarly work, and individualizing learning to support career goals.[11] Bridges includes three phases of education: Foundations 1 (years 1 and 2), Foundations 2 (core clerkships), and Career Launch (subinternships and electives).

The CMC is a longitudinal 15-month clinical skills and health systems course during Foundations 1 for first- and second-year medical students. The CMC curriculum is delivered in the classroom, in the simulation center, and at a variety of clinical sites known as microsystems. These clinical microsystems serve as small microcosms of three larger affiliated health systems (academic, county, and veterans). During the COVID-19 pandemic, from March to June 2020, small-group activities were converted to a purely virtual format, including standardized patient encounters via telemedicine. Microsystems work and health systems improvement activities continued virtually; in cases where this was not possible, students pivoted to new projects related to COVID-19. In the 2020 to 2021 academic year, students were able to return to in-person learning for essential activities, such as physical exam skills and certain microsystem activities.

Students participate in the CMC 1 day/week within longitudinal learning communities consisting of small groups of five or six students led by a physician faculty coach. One half-day of each week is focused on health systems improvement. The CMC health systems improvement curriculum focuses on specific improvement topics, interprofessional collaboration, and the development of a professional identity within complex teams and systems. Students work and learn directly with their coaches and members of the interprofessional team on a longitudinal project that addresses a problem in the microsystem. Fig. 8.1 illustrates an overview of the components of the CMC health systems improvement curriculum.

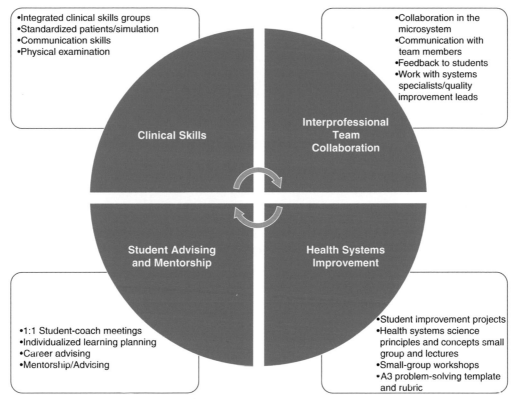

•Integrated clinical skills groups
•Standardized patients/simulation
•Communication skills
•Physical examination

•Collaboration in the
 microsystem
•Communication with
 team members
•Feedback to students
•Work with systems
 specialists/quality
 improvement leads

Clinical Skills

Interprofessional Team Collaboration

Student Advising and Mentorship

Health Systems Improvement

•1:1 Student-coach meetings
•Individualized learning planning
•Career advising
•Mentorship/Advising

•Student improvement projects
•Health systems science
 principles and concepts small
 group and lectures
•Small-group workshops
•A3 problem-solving template
 and rubric

Fig. 8.1 University of California, San Francisco, School of Medicine Clinical Microsystems Clerkship Health System Improvement Curricular Components.

Faculty Development

At UCSF, physician coaches guide early medical student learning of HSS. They are all clinician educator faculty, representing over 20 different medical specialties, who are competitively selected and financially supported to serve as mentors throughout medical school as well as teachers for the CMC curriculum. Coaches guide health systems improvement projects, mostly in small-group sessions at the clinical microsystem. Coaches are chosen for their commitment to medical student education. Many coaches do not have training or experience in HSS or quality improvement efforts prior to joining the CMC.

Faculty development is a cornerstone of professional development for coaches and helps to standardize the learning experience for students across all clinical sites. Fig. 8.2 illustrates the topics covered in faculty development, including HSS, project planning, and coaching skills. Content is delivered via weekly events, including large groups, small groups, and individual instruction. During the academic school year, weekly faculty development sessions cover the upcoming CMC curriculum activities in the next week and includes "just in time" announcements. Twice a year, all coaches attend a full day of faculty development sessions, including interactive small-group workshops and discussions on topics ranging from classroom activities, health systems improvement activities, mentoring, and career advising.

Eight months before the start of every academic year, coaches begin a detailed process to guide the development of quality improvement projects in preparation for student entry. As part of the health systems improvement preparation process, each coach meets with the CMC leadership team three to four times prior to the student's arrival and completes a project workbook detailing the project, including a metrics/data acquisition plan, list of the interprofessional team, and logistics on working in the microsystem.

Student Projects

Students are introduced to HSS concepts, including **Lean methodology**, through approximately 20 hours of foundational large-group didactics and small-group workshops prior to their project launch. Working and learning on their

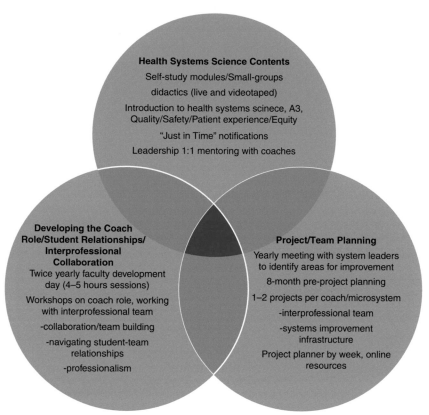

Fig. 8.2 University of California, San Francisco, School of Medicine Clinical Microsystems Clerkship Health Systems Improvement Faculty Development.

health systems improvement projects begins with a health system "immersion week," during which first-year medical students meet chief executive officers, shadow interprofessional clinicians, and listen to the stories of patients cared for in that health system. Boxes 8.1 to 8.4 highlight select student projects with student reflections on the process.

Throughout the remaining 15 months, the students track progress on their project using an adapted **Lean A3 template**, a standardized health care continuous improvement tool originally developed by and for the Toyota Motor Corporation to document and track improvements in manufacturing processes.[12,13] The CMC A3, adapted from the Lean A3, is a problem-solving tool and a document, originally based on the size of A3 paper (11 × 17 inches), to visually and graphically demonstrate and track the iterative process and progress of the student health systems improvement project over time. The CMC A3 includes the following components in order: (1) describe the problem, (2) current state (with process mapping and flowcharts), (3) target goal, (4) gap analysis—why the problem exists, (5) experiments/interventions description, (6) action plan, and

(7) study/reflect/next steps. Fig. 8.3 illustrates a CMC Lean A3 template.

While focus areas differ, all students participate actively in the systems improvement efforts using the same standard Lean systematic problem-solving approach, interact regularly with health system team members, and collaborate with other students to complete the project. Student groups work with their coach and interprofessional health care professionals—nurses, social workers, pharmacists, physical therapists, systems specialists, case managers, and others—in the microsystem. For their health system problem, students complete background research, process mapping, **gap analysis**, intervention(s) with **Plan-Do-Study-Act (PDSA) cycles**, measurement, evaluation, and reflections on lessons learned and project sustainability. All student project focus areas address local and national priority areas in quality improvement, patient safety, health equity, the patient experience, high value care, and access to care.

Examples of projects have included reducing readmissions to the inpatient psychiatry service to engaging patients in education around care after a concussion to developing a system to report patients with recurrent seizures to

---

BOX 8.1   Addressing Disparities in Hypertension Management

Project Description—Improving Hypertension Control for African Americans in Primary Care

In the primary care clinic, rates of uncontrolled hypertension were 41% among African American patients compared with 25.7% in other racial groups. The team's goal was to improve hypertension control* for African American patients over a 9-month period. Students developed and implemented an outreach telephone program to (1) schedule blood pressure check appointments, (2) understand patient perceptions of gaps, and (3) schedule follow-up office visits with a doctor or nurse to address needs and barriers.

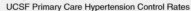

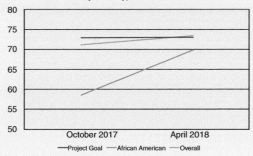

UCSF Primary Care Hypertension Control Rates

—Project Goal —African American —Overall

- **Overall, control rates increased by 10% and, for patients with uncontrolled hypertension, 38%.**
- **The program's hypertension control measurement criteria were adopted as a new methodology by the [institution].**

[Institution] Hypertension Control Rates

Lessons Learned/Value Added to the System

As we were doing our interprofessional interviews we learned that many nurses had patient panels whom they were following up with to monitor and counsel for their hypertension. It became clear to us through this QI project that nurses, physician assistants, and other interprofessional members are a valuable resource in understanding patient barriers and experiences in the health care process.

—Student team

---

* Definition of "controlled" blood pressure: systolic blood pressure below 140 mm Hg and diastolic blood pressure below 90 mm Hg for adults ages 18–59; a blood pressure reading below 140 mm Hg/90 mm Hg in adults ages 60–86 with diabetes mellitus; and a blood pressure reading below 150 mm Hg/90 mm Hg in adults ages 60–86 without diabetes mellitus

the department of motor vehicles. Table 8.1 includes a list of selected projects, health care systems (county, academic, veterans), interventions, and outcomes. Boxes 8.1 to 8.4 highlight several additional examples with a description, outcomes, impact to the system, and lessons learned from the students' perspective.

LEARNING GOALS

The goal of this health systems improvement activity is for students to apply a standard process to address a current problem in health care, work with an interprofessional team, and contribute value for the patients and clinicians of their clinical **microsystem**. Sample curricular learning objectives for students include (1) identify how microsystem improvement work supports organizational, regulatory, payment, public reporting, or internal quality goals; (2) apply knowledge and communication skills for effective

interprofessional collaboration in health care; and (3) seek, reflect on, share, and incorporate feedback and data from the clinical workplace.

TECHNIQUES TO ASSESS LEARNERS

Student assessment includes a combination of strategies to allow learners to demonstrate their HSS knowledge and skills, including (1) the Quality Improvement Knowledge Application Tool-Revised (QIKAT-R), (2) completion of a student group CMC Lean A3 document at several timepoints during the CMC, and (3) individualized interprofessional team member feedback. The timeline for these assessments is shown in Fig. 8.4.

Twice a year, students individually complete the QIKAT-R, a validated knowledge test on quality improvement knowledge.[14] The QIKAT presents a clinical scenario with a systems problem and has three-part open-ended questions: (1) identifying the

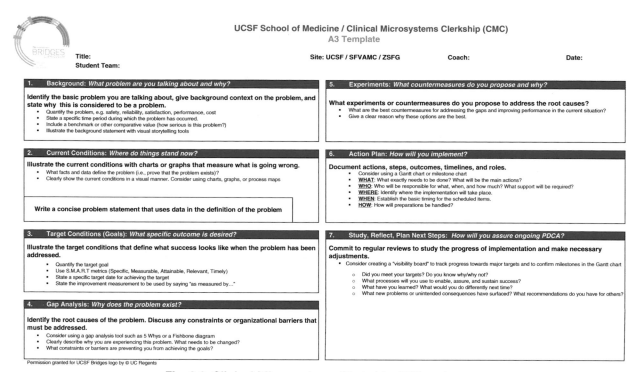

Fig. 8.3 Clinical Microsystems Clerkship A3 Template.

aim by writing an aim statement, (2) listing the measures used to assess the problem, and (3) describing one experiment/intervention to test what may address the aim.

The UCSF-adapted CMC Lean A3 problem-solving tool is completed by student groups and assessed at several checkpoints during the CMC using a rubric developed by the CMC leadership team. Using rubrics for the QIKAT and the A3, coaches and CMC leadership assess each student (via QIKAT) and student group (via the Lean A3) as having "met" or "not met" expectations. In the spring of the first year, students identify an interprofessional health care professional (not a physician) from whom they receive feedback about strengths and areas for improvement. Results for the QIKAT, Lean A3, and interprofessional feedback are shared with the student on an online "dashboard" accessible to the students and their coaches. At the end of the 15-month period, student teams create and present a poster during a quality improvement symposium.

EVALUATION PROCEDURES

Program evaluation includes both qualitative and quantitative measures. Overall student satisfaction is high, averaging 4.60 on a scale 1 (low) to 5 (high) over the past 4 years. Students described learning of health system teams

and processes immediately after the end of the curriculum, followed by the application of these systems improvement concepts in their clerkship years. Students have consistently rated the CMC and their relationship with their coaches as one of the most formative experiences in their medical education. Several years into the program, students now report presenting their health systems improvement project outcomes at local, regional, and national professional society meetings; as part of their residency applications; and as peer-reviewed manuscripts.

Value Added to the Health Care System: CMC Project Examples and Outcomes

From 2016 to 2020, a total of 617 students participated in 218 health system improvement projects across three health systems in 165 microsystems. The projects range from interventions that address patient safety (e.g., reducing surgical site infections) to screening and prevention (e.g., increasing vaccination rates); to addressing the patient experience (e.g., improving education on HIV pre-exposure prophylaxis); to fostering health equity (e.g., improving postpartum care for at-risk women). Table 8.1 highlights a selection of the projects completed and in progress from 2016 to 2020 and Fig. 8.3 includes an example of a CMC A3 template.

BOX 8.2 Managing Postdischarge Opioids on a Surgical Service

Project Description—Postoperative Outpatient Opioid Prescription and Disposal After Minimally Invasive Gynecology Oncology Surgery

To address the over-prescription, overuse, and potential waste of opioids in the postoperative setting, the team worked collaboratively with the [institution]. Gynecology Oncology Enhanced Recovery Pathway (ERAS) to identify safe opioid prescribing practices and disposal. A multimodal intervention included (1) a standardized electronic prescribing dot phrase for oxycodone #20 5-mg tablets on discharge, (2) educational campaign for providers, and (3) discharge instructions for patients on disposal kiosks and mail-back programs.

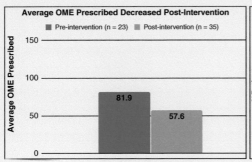

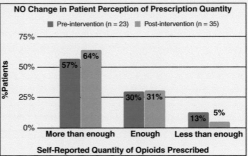

Pre- and post-intervention cohorts were similar with regards to race, ethnicity, age, BMI, preferred language, and distribution of the type of minimally invasive surgeries performed

- **Decreased OME prescribed at discharge by 30%**
- **No change in patient perception of pain control after hospitalization**
- **Written discharge instructions did not increase knowledge on safe disposal options**
  OME, Oral morphine equivalent.

Lessons Learned/Value Added to the System

We gained substantial useful local knowledge regarding our gynecology oncology microsystem. We learned about the local resources for disposing of opioids. We also learned about opportunities and barriers in the department that either facilitate or hinder long-term change. This includes the constant change of residents, fellows, and providers, along with the cohesive teamwork and support throughout the department.

— **Student team**

TABLE 8.1 Selected UCSF Clinical Microsystem Clerkship Student Projects 2016–2020

Category	Microsystem	Project	Health System	Outcomes/Value Added to the System
Quality Improvement/ Patient Safety	Hospital/Pediatric Nursery	Identify secondhand smoke (SHS) exposure in the neonatal inpatient setting	County	Developed a template to screen and document SHS for all discharged patients.
Quality Improvement/ Patient Safety	Hospital/PACU	Improving prophylaxis of postoperative nausea and vomiting	Academic	Created a PACU order set to provide additional antiemetic options. Reduced the use of repeat antiemetic orders from 41.9% to 32.1%.

(Continued)

TABLE 8.1   Selected UCSF Clinical Microsystem Clerkship Student Projects 2016–2020—cont'd

Category	Microsystem	Project	Health System	Outcomes/Value Added to the System
Health Equity/ Access to Care	Family Birth Center	Improving postpartum care for women with open CPS cases	County	Assembled "Plan of Safe Care Collaborative," a multidisciplinary support system for patients at risk of CPS referral spanning the prenatal, intrapartum, and postpartum periods, and provides holistic support for patients at risk of a CPS referral.
Health Equity/ Access to Care	Ambulatory Clinic	Establishing a new interprofessional trans health clinic	Veterans	Decreased the average wait time to hormone initiation from 91 to 14 days. Developed a website and orientation packet for new patients. Collaborated with an endocrinologist, social workers, psychologists, and primary care providers to establish a new trans health clinic.
High Value Care	Hospital/ Neurosurgery Unit	Reduction of postoperative dexamethasone in craniotomy patients	Academic	Developed an EHR order set for a no-default option for dexamethasone dosing. Reduced postoperative dexamethasone to 4 mg twice daily from 5% to 20% over a 12-month period.
High Value Care	Hospital/Pediatric Service	Albuterol weaning guideline for pediatric asthma patients	County	Implemented an evidence-based guideline to wean albuterol. Over a 4-month period decreased LOS from 2.1 days to 1.2 days (43% decrease).
Patient Experience	Skilled Nursing Facility	Nonpharmacologic pain control interventions in the community living center	Veterans	Created a templated EHR note to include the option to refer patients for cognitive behavioral therapy (CBT). Increased documentation to offer CBT from 18% to 80% for all patients with moderate to severe chronic pain over a 3-month period.
Patient Experience	Lung Transplant Clinic	Reducing stress and promoting wellness in posttransplant caregivers	Academic	Distributed high yield and low cost resources for caregivers to practice mindfulness and self-care in a "blue binder," rated as useful to >70% of caregivers.

CPS, Child protective services; *EHR*, electronic health record; *ICU*, intensive care unit; *LOS*, length of stay; *PACU*, post-acute care unit; *UCSF*, University of California, San Francisco.

BOX 8.3 Improving Quality and the Patient Experience in the Hospital

Project Description—Improving Inpatient Sleep: Reducing Nighttime Meds

Sleep deprivation is a common occurrence in the hospital and can contribute to increased mortality, morbidity, impaired healing, and delirium. The "Dream Team" identified several factors that led to increased interruptions at night for patients assigned to sleep promotion vital signs (vital signs taken only during the day). On average, ~2 medications were ordered and administered overnight, thus disrupting optimal sleep hours. Acetaminophen accounted for 11% of those medications. The intervention included an educational campaign to retime medication orders and an electronic ordering default for acetaminophen to every 8 hours (instead of every 6 hours).

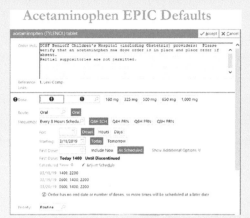

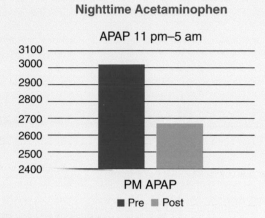

- **Team successfully launched an electronic prescribing order default for acetaminophen.**
- **Nighttime acetaminophen administration (between 11 pm and 5 am) decreased by > 50% over a 6-month period.**

Lessons Learned/Value Added to the System

Quality improvement relies on a four-legged stool approach for success: education, culture change, informatics change, audit/feedback.

— Student team

Boxes 8.1 to 8.4 highlight four student projects that exemplify the diversity of problems students addressed as value-added members to the system and the students' responses to their experience. In each of these examples, students were embedded into the system improvement activities on a regular basis, working directly with an interprofessional team and their coach. Each student group had team and individual roles and responsibilities and were value added in different ways, ultimately resulting in a change to the system.

RESOURCES NEEDED

The design phase of the UCSF Bridges curriculum began in 2012 to develop "collaboratively expert physicians" who provide safe, high-quality, and equitable care within interprofessional systems. In 2013, UCSF School of Medicine received a $1 million grant from the American Medical Association for the proposal "Bridges to High-Quality Health Care Curriculum," to support the revamp of the medical school curriculum. Spearheaded by Catherine Lucey, MD, vice dean for education at the UCSF School of Medicine, the curriculum redesign included a new funding infrastructure in partnership among deans, chairs, and medical education to support the core education staff and faculty. "We are committed to designing this curriculum so that our students, from the time they begin medical school, are prepared to add value to the clinical sites in which they are learning."[15] UCSF School of Medicine leadership, including all the deans, were involved in every facet of development and implementation, from retreats and working groups to curriculum details and recruiting faculty as coaches. The CMC's goals and objectives for the health systems improvement curriculum were built on the original call to change how medical education was taught to future physicians.[16]

The CMC health systems improvement curriculum was developed by CMC curriculum leaders (n = 8), implemented by a team of full-time medical education staff (n = 6), and delivered to the students by physician faculty coaches (n = 50) funded for 1 day/week. Multiple additional educational and clinical teams support the curricular and coaching programs. The financial investment is committed by the school of medicine dean and all department chairs; this central high-intensity teaching fund is managed by the education dean. Deans and chairs view this investment positively due to the involvement of faculty from a variety of departments, the shared belief in supporting

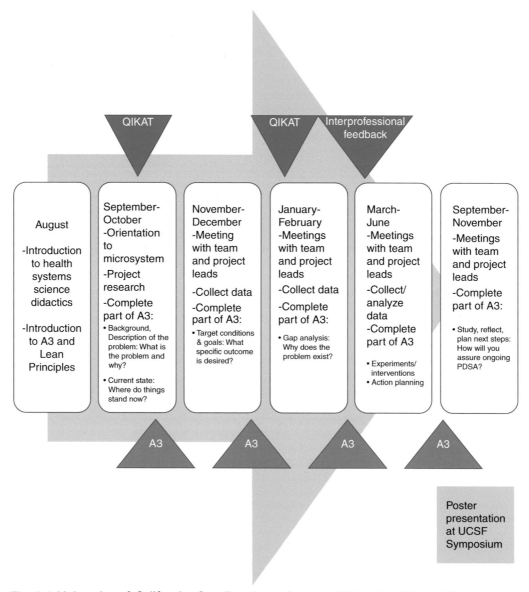

Fig. 8.4 University of California, San Francisco, School of Medicine Clinical Microsystems Clerkship Health Systems Improvement Curriculum and Assessment Timeline. *PDSA*, Plan-Do-Study-Act; *QIKAT*, Quality Improvement Knowledge Application Tool; *UCSF*, University of California, San Francisco.

BOX 8.4   Alerts During Infectious Outbreaks at a Skilled Nursing Facility

Project Description—Development of an Infection Control Protocol for a Skilled Nursing Facility
In previous years, a skilled nursing facility had experienced several infectious disease outbreaks, including norovirus, influenza, and rhinovirus. In each instance, lapses in communication across systems were attributed to delays in containment. This project focused on identifying and clarifying a protocol to alert providers and respond to a documented or potential outbreak. The team worked with infection control, environmental management services, dietitians, physicians, and nurse managers to educate and disseminate the protocol, including a reporting system and next steps.

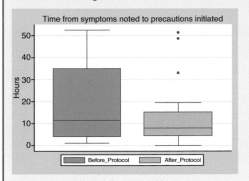

- **Protocol decreased the mean response time from first noted symptoms to the initiation of precautions during an outbreak by 31%, from 20.1 to 13.8 hours**

Lessons Learned/Value Added to the System
We learned about the importance of understanding the different stakeholders involved in preventing infectious outbreaks, particularly stakeholders not traditionally considered part of the care team, such as cleaning and food services staff. We also learned about the multiple different communication modalities (email, phone, charts, etc.), and the importance of acknowledging each stakeholder's preferred communication method.

— **Student team**

---

educators and the education mission, as well as the vision of improving today's health systems while equipping our physicians-in-training with skills needed to care for their future patients.

Physician coaches were selected based on their outstanding experience as clinician-educators, interest in working with medical students, and motivation to teach HSS while improving care in their microsystems. Prior to the start of the CMC, over 75% coaches did not have any previous training, experience, or expertise in HSS. This gap highlighted the need for a faculty development program to provide a longitudinal and continuous experience for coaches as health systems improvement educators and to support their professional development.

IMPLEMENTATION HISTORY AND STRATEGIES EMPLOYED

In anticipation of the launch of the UCSF Bridges Curriculum in 2016, curricular leaders carried out multiple rounds of design and pilots. Starting in 2012, institutional education and clinical leaders across three health systems gathered to articulate a vision for engaging students in HSS. Starting in 2013,

the prior version of the preclerkship clinical skills curriculum began constructing the building blocks that would serve as the foundation of the new health systems curriculum. In 2014, faculty in three different microsystems (rheumatology, cardiology, and hospital medicine) conducted an early experiential health systems curriculum pilot as a two-month elective with 10 medical students. This elective identified these best practices for the subsequent Bridge's health systems improvement curriculum: (1) a longitudinal faculty coach who provides guidance and expertise, (2) the choice of projects that are meaningful to and supported by health system leadership, (3) opportunities for students to learn from the interprofessional team, and (4) a concurrent HSS curricula for both faculty coaches and students that aligns with health system practices. The CMC successfully launched in 2016 and continues to evolve each year based on real-time evaluation data.

KEY ADVICE FOR FEASIBILITY AND SUSTAINABILITY

Recent literature describes six major themes for incorporating students in value-added roles: educational value; value added to the microsystem; mentor time and microsystem capacity; student engagement; relationships among students, the microsystem, and the school; and longitudinal continuity.[17] In the process of designing and launching a new early medical student curriculum focused on experiential health systems improvement, we have uncovered five best practices for feasibility, effectiveness, and sustainability.

First, resources and time must be allocated to teach a project-based health systems improvement curriculum, and it must be supported by leadership. The resources should include (1) funded teaching and mentoring time for physician coaches (0.2 FTE or 1 day/week), supported by their department and department chair to be away from clinical activities; (2) faculty development to ensure that coaches incorporate the curriculum content and delivery; and (3) dedicated time in the preclerkship medical school curriculum for health systems improvement (1 day/week) during all instructional weeks.

Second, another key to the success is the integration of longitudinal health systems improvement into the larger curricular and assessment frameworks. Students see this required curriculum on their integrated school calendar, along with clinical skills and foundational science sessions. Student assessments (i.e., the QIKAT, A3, and interprofessional feedback) are requirements for passing the integrated courses, such as foundational science examinations. This requirement helps to frame the importance and value of health systems improvement as a core part of the student's educational experience.

Third, the importance of creating a partnership between the school of medicine and affiliated health systems cannot be overstated. This partnership goes both ways, and each partner benefits from it. When students are truly and authentically embedded in health systems improvement activities over a period of time and can observe the effects and outcomes of their efforts, then there is a sense of ownership and empowerment over the work.

Fourth, successful student integration into health systems improvement activities requires a considerable amount of intentional, early steady planning within a context of continuous improvement on the part of the curriculum leaders and the coaches. Coaches and curriculum leaders meet to develop the student projects, meet with health system leaders to align priorities, select a meaningful problem, identify data streams, and assemble an interprofessional team. These efforts require time and expertise.

Finally, celebrating successes with high-visibility events is important to the sustainability of health systems improvement. One of the key domains of quality improvement is communication and dissemination—the system will not know that the work is being done unless it is shared. All students demonstrate their value to the health care systems by showing their project outcomes at a poster symposium including health system leaders and medical education deans. Every year, four student groups are invited to share more details in oral presentations at a highly visible event in the presence of all the school of medicine deans and leadership from UCSF and UCSF-affiliated sites, including the chief operating officers, chief quality officers, and chief medical officers.

FACULTY REFLECTIONS

Working with students in the CMC has been a highlight of my career at UCSF. As an educator, I think it is both incredible, and so important, that the school of medicine has committed time and resources to invite students into my clinical world of primary care, see how we provide care for patients, and from there, engage in a quality improvement project. As a clinician, I've loved how working with students in the CMC has also led me to partner with my division's clinical and quality improvement leaders to positively impact patient care. Whether working with students to improve naloxone co-prescription rates for patients on chronic opiates, reduce polypharmacy for patients over 65, or improve advanced care planning documentation for limited English proficiency patients, I believe that there were several keys to our success. First, students are engaged and eager to make a difference. They are not simply learning an approach to QI, but actually applying it to a microsystem and patient population that they have early experience in. Second, the CMC is an 18-month experience. This degree of longitudinality really allows students time to immerse in the microsystem and thoughtfully conduct their needs assessment, carry out their gap analysis, employ an intervention, and assess the impact of that intervention. Third, the CMC provides ample faculty resources. From initial planning meetings and regular check-ins to faculty development on HSS topics, the program sets us up to be confident in our skills and succeed in guiding our students through their projects. Through my role in the CMC, I feel like I have learned alongside my students and advanced my own skillset in HSS, all while developing incredible relationships with my students and colleagues.

—Leslie Sheu, MD,
Department of Medicine,
Division of General Internal Medicine,
Medical Student Coach

STUDENT REFLECTIONS

My project was focused on reducing the incidence of delirium in the hospital. With my QI partner, I helped to create a feasible delirium precautions audit that nurses could perform quickly. The impact of our project focused on providing hospital staff with an easy-to-use, reliable, and efficient audit tool that could be used to trace implementation of delirium precautions in the hospital. I learned that health systems science allows everyone working in the clinical ecosystem to propose changes to improve patient care or the provider experience. As a student, I had the protected time to help determine the barriers to implementing change, enabling me to perform a complete analysis. Quality improvement work is imperative for medical students because it teaches an evidenced-based method to problem solving that students can implement in all health care settings and across patient populations. Our patients face numerous barriers associated with public health and health care systems in this country. By learning how to address problems as a function of the system, as a 3rd-year student I can help patients alter the systems in their own lives to improve their own health outcomes.

—Christopher Johnson,
Third-Year Medical Student

CONCLUSION

With years of planning, investment of resources, and a spirit of continuous improvement, the experience at UCSF demonstrates that even early medical students can engage in meaningful, longitudinal value-added roles in health systems improvement. Funding for faculty time, integration of health systems improvement as core curriculum, partnership between the school of medicine and health system leaders, intentional early planning, and celebrations of project outcomes were key to feasibility and success. Future directions include further examination of long-term sustainability, clear definitions of value from the health system perspective, and added focus on improving urgent gaps, such as health equity and disparities.

REFERENCES

1. Irby DM, Cooke M, O'Brien BC. Calls for reform of medical education by the Carnegie Foundation for the Advancement of Teaching: 1910 and 2010. *Acad Med*. 2010;85(2):220–227. https://doi.org/10.1097/ACM.0b013e3181c88449.

2. Gonzalo JD, Lucey C, Wolpaw T, Chang A. Value-added clinical systems learning roles for medical students that transform education and health: a guide for building partnerships between medical schools and health systems. *Acad Med*. 2017;92:602–607. https://doi.org/10.1097/ACM.0000000000001346.

3. Grumbach K, Lucey CR, Claiborne Johnston S. Transforming from centers of learning to learning health systems: the challenge for academic health centers. *JAMA*. 2014;311(11):1109–1110. https://doi.org/10.1001/jama.2014.705.

4. Bergh AM, Bac M, Hugo J, Sandars J. "Making a difference"—Medical students' opportunities for transformational change in health care and learning through quality improvement projects. *BMC Med Educ*. 2016;11(16):171. https://doi.org/10.1186/s12909-016-0694-1.

5. Lave J, Wenger E. *Situated Learning: Legitimate Peripheral Participation*. Cambridge, MA: Cambridge University Press; 1991.

6. Cruess RL, Cruess SR, Steinert Y. Medicine as a community of practice: implications for medical education. *Acad Med*. 2018;93:185–191. https://doi.org/10.1097/ACM.0000000000001826.

7. Dornan T, Boshuizen H, King N, Sherpbier A. Experience-based learning: a model linking processes and outcomes of medical students' workplace learning. *Med Educ*. 2007;41(1):84–91. https://doi.org/10.1111/j.1365-2929.2006.02652.x.

8. Dornan T. Workplace learning. *Perspect Med Educ*. 2012;1(1):15–23. https://doi.org/10.1007/s40037-012-0005-4.

9. Gonzalo JD, Ogrinc G. Health systems science: the "broccoli" of undergraduate medical education. *Acad Med*. 2019;94:1425–1432. https://doi.org/10.1097/ACM.0000000000002815.

10. Burnett E, Davey P, Gray N, Tully V, Breckenridge J. Medical students as agents of change: a qualitative exploratory study *BMJ Open Qual*. 2018;7:e000420. https://doi.org/10.1136/bmjoq-2018-000420.

11. UCSF School of Medicine. Bridges Curriculum. https://meded.ucsf.edu/bridges-curriculum. Accessed 16.12.20.

12. Jimmerson C. *A3 Problem Solving for Healthcare: A Practical Method for Eliminating Waste*. New York, NY: Productivity Press; 2007.

13. Chakravorty SS. Process improvement: using Toyota's A3 reports. *Qual Manag J*. 2009;16(4):7–26. https://doi.org/10.1080/10686967.2009.11918247.

14. Singh MK, Ogrinc G, Cox KR, et al. The Quality Improvement Knowledge Application Tool Revised (QIKAT-R). *Acad Med*. 2014;89(10):1386–1391. https://doi.org/10.1097/ACM.0000000000000456.

15. Norris, J. AMA Awards $1M to UCSF to Transform Physician Training. UCSF website. https://www.ucsf.edu/news/2013/06/106731/ama-awards-1m-ucsf-transform-physician-training. Accessed 16.12.20.

16. American Medical Association *Creating a Community of Innovation*. Chicago, IL: American Medical Association; 2017.

https://www.ama-assn.org/sites/ama-assn.org/files/corp/media-browser/public/about-ama/ace-monograph-interactive_0.pdf. Accessed 16.12.20.

17. Gonzalo JD, Graaf D, Ahluwalia A, Wolpaw DR, Thompson BM. A practical guide for implementing and maintaining value-added clinical systems learning roles for medical students using a diffusion of innovations framework. *Adv Health Sci Educ Theory Pract.* 2018;23(4):699–720. https://doi.org/10.1007/s10459-018-9822-5.

9

Plan-Do-Study-Act: Vanderbilt University School of Medicine

Heather A. Ridinger, Jennifer K. Green, and Anderson Spickard III

LEARNING OBJECTIVES

1. Describe the Vanderbilt University School of Medicine approach to teaching quality improvement.
2. Outline key outcome measures from the Foundations of Healthcare Delivery Quality Improvement courses.
3. List lessons learned and key advice for feasibility and sustainability.

OUTLINE

CHAPTER SUMMARY

In this chapter, we summarize the approach that Vanderbilt University School of Medicine has taken in teaching and implementing individual or paired quality improvement (QI) projects for all third-year medical students. We highlight curricular design, implementation strategies, resources needed, and key lessons learned. QI is included as part of a larger 4-year longitudinal course called Foundations of Healthcare Delivery (FHD), which teaches students throughout all years the core content of health systems science. QI projects are student driven in a clinical site of their choosing. Three QI courses are offered monthly; students have 15 months to complete each of the three courses alongside their other clinical requirements. The QI courses are administered by two faculty block directors with QI expertise and overseen by three FHD course directors. In addition, each student project is assisted by a faculty project sponsor who is a clinic stakeholder and assists students in accessing data and implementing the changes. Student projects are often small in scope and are designed to prioritize student learning over meeting institutional QI needs. Here, we summarize the findings for our course since its inception in 2014 and provide a detailed analysis of the QI projects completed within the last two academic years. We conclude that instruction in QI, along with the support and accountability to perform QI projects, can help students become change agents who make small but important and impactful adjustments to the clinical microsystems in which they work and learn.

INTRODUCTION

In response to a call for increased quality and safety training for medical graduates, Vanderbilt University School of Medicine conducted a needs assessment. Staff determined there was mounting concern that traditional training models were not meeting the needs of a dynamic 21st-century health care system.[1] With this goal in mind, Vanderbilt underwent a curricular revision called Curriculum 2.0 beginning in 2012. Institutional leadership envisioned a curriculum that incorporated health systems science (HSS)[2-4] as a key component in an integrated system of learning. For this purpose, we designed the Foundations of Healthcare Delivery (FHD) course as a required, longitudinal 4-year course that aims to teach students the breadth of HSS while integrating those sciences with clinical care. We conceived FHD around the conceptual framework of the **National Academy of Medicine aims of quality health care**: safe, timely, effective, efficient, equitable, and patient centered.[5-7] The overall goals of the longitudinal FHD course are to (1) prepare professionals with systems-level skills necessary to provide care that is safe, timely, effective, efficient, equitable, and patient centered; (2) integrate health systems knowledge with clinical care; and (3) cultivate respectful professionals.

FHD curricular content and structure varies in each of the years of medical training. Medical students begin in their first year embedded in a single-continuity **clinical microsystem**,[8] attending a single clinic for one afternoon each week during the first year, in which they learn the structure and function of the interprofessional clinical team and patient population. Students also learn principles of medication safety, social determinants of health, and behavioral health change. Students progress from this continuity clinical microsystem to learning skills for effective care delivery in **mesosystems** and **macrosystems** in subsequent years. Second-year students on core clinical clerkship learn key skills related to the mesosystem of the hospital, including patient safety incident reporting, transitions of care, settings of care, high-value care, advocacy, and clinical informatics/health information technology. During the immersion phase (years 3–4), FHD content relates to macrosystems and systems improvements: **quality improvement (QI)**, patient safety risk identification and event analyses, population and public health, interprofessional education, and health care economics and policy.

DESCRIPTION OF FOUNDATIONS OF HEALTHCARE DELIVERY QUALITY IMPROVEMENT COURSES AT VANDERBILT UNIVERSITY SCHOOL OF MEDICINE

Curricular Design

The FHD QI courses are taught during the third year of medical school. As with all other FHD courses, the QI courses focus on experiential workplace-based learning[9] by enabling students to plan and enact a QI project in a clinical setting of their choice. The course didactics use the **Institute for Healthcare Improvement (IHI) Model for Improvement** as a conceptual framework.[10,11] Students are encouraged to engage with the stakeholders in the clinical setting. The goals of the course are intended to assist students in understanding and experiencing the process of improvement. The educational opportunity and autonomy of students is prioritized over expectations for process outcomes or meeting institutional QI needs. Students are encouraged to find small manageable projects in a clinical setting that is meaningful to them. These projects often align with the students' future career interests. Thus, projects are often small in scope and completed by individuals or pairs of students. In this way, students assume the role of **change agents**. By designing the curriculum around the needs of the students rather than the institution or clinical setting, students gain flexibility to not only find a project that is meaningful to them but for which they have optimal control over the planning, execution, and outcome.

Course Logistics

The FHD course began with the inaugural class in 2012; we implemented the first QI curriculum for third-year students during the 2014 to 2015 academic year. The QI curriculum involves three sequential month-long courses: QI 1 to 3 taught by two faculty block directors and overseen by three FHD course directors. The QI courses are designed to be taken sequentially (although not necessarily in consecutive months) as each course walks students stepwise through their QI projects. Each of the three courses is approximately 20 hours of curricular work. The format involves asynchronous learning wherein students review course readings and complete specific modules on the IHI Open School platform and face-to-face course meetings with faculty block directors. Students can enroll in these QI courses along with a clinical or elective rotation. Students have Tuesday afternoons as protected time to work on FHD requirements during months that they are enrolled. Students must complete each of the three QI courses within a 15-month period (September of the third year through November of the fourth year). A maximum of 20 students can register in each of the three courses, which are offered monthly. Fig. 9.1 depicts an example student schedule with FHD QI courses scheduled concurrently with the third year Research Immersion course.

Each student chooses a clinical microsystem and affiliated faculty project sponsor who helps the student through the process of planning and enacting the QI project. The project sponsor is often a clinician in the clinical site and serves as the microsystem expert and student champion. Faculty sponsors are not paid for their participation in the QI program but can submit their time for Part 4 Maintenance of Certification (MOC) Credit as an incentive. The faculty block directors are salary supported for their work in the QI course. Block directors have QI expertise. Their responsibilities include guiding the course and providing instruction, offering feedback on student-led projects, and submitting final grades. All students complete an electronic poster describing their project. Students present their completed projects to peers in a classroom setting. Additionally, interested students can submit their poster for presentation at an annual Vanderbilt University School of Medicine QI Symposium held during their fourth year.

LEARNING GOALS

Learning goals for the FHD QI courses are designed to help students through the process of planning and executing their QI project and include:

1. Understand the need for QI and patient safety in health care to be conducted in a thoughtful, organized, and structured framework, using the IHI Model for Improvement to systematically enact change.
2. Utilize QI methods to identify gaps and/or deviations in system-based processes that lead to inefficiencies, waste, drift, ineffective care, and/or inequitable care.
3. Recognize the need for a multidisciplinary team and the right stakeholders when starting and implementing a QI project.
4. Differentiate between QI and research methodologies.

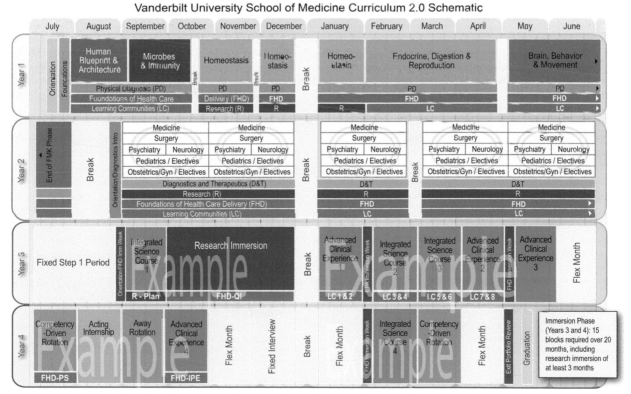

Fig. 9.1 Example of Vanderbilt University Medical Student Schedule.

5. Create and enact a measurement plan based on qualitative data obtained during the clinical problem assessment phase and determine the feasibility of the plan.

6. Create a "SMART" (**s**pecific, **m**easurable, **a**chievable, **r**elevant, **t**ime-bound) aim statement based on both qualitative and quantitative analysis of the clinical problem.

7. Devise a system-based plan to mitigate the identified clinical problem using the IHI Model for Improvement.

8. Summarize the findings of a QI project and reflect on ways to implement, sustain, and spread change.

9. Understand the methods and value of using run charts to enhance understanding of whether tested changes are leading to improvement.

10. Describe cultural barriers to enacting change, strategies to motivate health care providers to be change agents, and factors to consider when spreading change to other clinical settings.

TECHNIQUES TO ASSESS LEARNERS

The three QI courses are graded on an honors/high pass/pass/fail grading system. Vanderbilt University School of Medicine is a competency-based medical education[10] program; as such, all students are assessed in a criterion-based approach. All students who meet the criteria for honors receive that grade. The course grades are composed of a knowledge assessment and project-related assignments. Student knowledge is assessed by an end course multiple choice question tool created by course faculty and derived from QI concepts covered in the IHI modules. The QI projects are broken down into discrete assignments to assist students' progression through the project. Each assignment has established criteria available to students as grading rubrics upon which a student's score is based. Formative qualitative feedback from faculty block directors help guide students by incorporating feedback into the next steps of the project.

EVALUATION PROCEDURES

Program evaluation uses a comprehensive and systematic approach to determine a program's effectiveness and identify areas for improvement.[12] Kirkpatrick's four-level program evaluation model provides a framework for understanding and classifying a variety of outcomes.[13] In this model, each level categorizes programmatic outcomes into increasingly complex measurements of a program's overall impact on learners and on society. The levels are described as (1) learner satisfaction or reaction to the program, (2) measures of learning, (3) changes in learner behavior, and (4) the program's impact on the institution

or community. Here, we describe outcomes from the QI courses using available programmatic evaluation data in an attempt to address each of the levels of the Kirkpatrick framework. Available data includes course evaluations (student impact), analysis of QI projects (measures of learning), and faculty feedback (impact on the institution and patient care).

Course Evaluations

Students complete an anonymous course evaluation after finishing the series of QI courses for the purpose of program evaluation and continuous improvement. The course evaluation is administered electronically by the Office of Evaluation and Assessment and is reviewed by course directors, administrators, and the Standing Assessment Committee, which includes a student course reviewer. Here, we review course evaluation data from academic years 2017 to 2018 and 2018 to 2019.

Overall, students value learning the process of QI, but they may differ on the ideal way to learn it. Most students favor learning QI by engaging in a hands-on project compared with learning content from didactics, although a minority of students would have preferred instead to simply observe QI projects at the medical center.

Students indicated that they had adequate time to devote to their QI projects during the course. They were uniformly pleased to have an opportunity to work with faculty sponsors in a clinical setting of their choosing and were grateful to be able to independently seek out and find a project that aligned with their interests or career goals. Students commented on the attentiveness to their scheduling needs by structuring the course with minimal in-class time, favoring independent protected time to work on projects. Students who worked in pairs on a project (29% of projects) were supportive of this option. Some students found it difficult to complete a QI project in the 3-month time frame, noting that they felt stressed or forced to complete a project on what seemed like an unnatural timeline. Similarly, students noted that assignment deadlines required flexibility when projects took unexpected turns, requiring them to adjust the project or regroup with faculty or stakeholders.

Course evaluation data revealed that knowledge assessments appeared to be misaligned with the information provided in the readings and modules. One student commented on the need to ensure that the assessments "don't test obscure details of the IHI modules [but] rather assess true understanding of the relevant topics." After revisions, this improved the following academic year (2018–2019). Students found the IHI didactics useful.

The most consistently identified area of improvement was the need for frequent and timely faculty feedback to allow for rapid-cycle improvement of students' projects.

In both academic years, students reported that a mere 50% received formative mid-course feedback crucial to their progression in the project. Many students reported that building a coalition and getting buy-in from stakeholders was one of the most challenging parts of the process for them, often leading to failed interventions or difficulty with sustainability. A few students (13%) did not feel that QI was a valuable part of their education or future career; one student expressed feeling that student QI projects were meant to help the medical center rather than further the students' education.

Among graduating students, 63% reported that they were asked about or talked about their QI project during one or more of their residency interviews. More than half of students "agreed" or "strongly agreed" that their completed QI project improved their competitiveness during the residency application process. This was especially true if students viewed their project as being successful or of good quality. Most students (85%) reported that they were "likely" or "very likely" to use the skills learned in the course in their future career. Learning the process of QI was the most valuable part of the course. While some students reported that their QI projects "did not work," others recognized that they were now able to evaluate the current state of their project and improve it. When asked about what completing a QI project taught them, one student commented, "I can be an agent of change to improve health systems."

Overall, course evaluation data supports that students overwhelmingly value learning the QI process and the majority prefer an active learning approach by completing a student-driven QI project in a clinical area of their choosing. Frequent and timely feedback from faculty is a key driver of student success and satisfaction. If projects are viewed as successful, students are more likely to recognize the value of the QI learning process on their residency application and future careers.

Analysis of Student-Driven Quality Improvement Projects

Since the course's inception in 2014 through 2019, students have completed 187 student-led QI projects across a variety of clinical sites, including in the medical center, the community, and student-led free clinics. We analyzed student QI project posters completed during the last two academic years (2017–2018 and 2018–2019, n = 95). Sixty-one projects (64%) were in the outpatient setting, 33 (35%) were in the inpatient setting, and 1 was both inpatient and outpatient. Seventeen (18%) of the QI projects were completed at the Shade Tree Clinic, Vanderbilt's student-run free clinic; 10 (11%) in other primary care settings; 14 (15%) in surgical subspecialty settings; 7 (7%) in the emergency department (ED); and 6 (6%) in intensive care.

Table 9.1 provides a description of the outcomes from student-led QI projects. The projects fell into one of four

TABLE 9.1   Analysis of Student-Driven QI Projects, 2017–2019

Project Type and Definition	Number of Projects	Average Outcome Score (0–2, SD)	Average Impact Score (0–2, SD)	Average Total Score (0–4, SD)
Patient Education: Projects aiming to provide education directed at patients or patient family/caregivers; no measurement on impact on care	18	1.22 (0.75)	0.64 (0.38)	1.81 (0.94)
Provider Education: Projects aiming to provide education directed at providers; no measurement on impact on care	12	1.33 (0.75)	0.71 (0.40)	2.04 (0.94)
Systems Redesign: Projects designed to improve patient flow, timeliness, streamline existing procedures or processes	35	1.10 (0.75)	1.00 (0.59)	2.06 (1.17)
Patient Care: Projects designed to improve patient care, including closing quality gaps and adherence to existing quality guidelines	30	1.12 (0.76)	0.88 (0.57)	1.95 (1.21)
Total	**95**	**1.16 (0.74)**	**0.86 (0.54)**	**1.97 (1.10)**

QI, Quality improvement.

project types depending on their stated aim or intervention: patient education, provider education, system redesign, and patient care. To determine the relative impact of these projects, two independent faculty experts scored each project using a 4-point scale, including 2 points for outcome (whether they did not meet [0 points], partially met [1 point], or fully met [2 points] their aim) and 2 points for impact (little to no impact [0 points], some impact [1 point], meaningful impact [2 points]). Projects with small sample sizes, education interventions that did not measure behaviors or learning retention, and interventions that did not produce changes in system processes or outcomes were assigned lower impact scores. In contrast, projects given higher impact scores demonstrated measurable improvements in system processes and outcomes, especially when the change was sustainable. Table 9.1 shows averaged scores from two reviewers (inter-rater reliability was 0.76).

From analyzing the QI projects in aggregate, we conclude that student projects are frequently small in scope and thus, outcomes are partially met with a moderate degree of variability. Students who choose system redesign and patient care projects tend to produce more meaningful or sustainable changes, as evidenced by higher impact scores. Impact scores among patient education projects on average are lower when compared with the other types, perhaps in part because students did not collect outcome measures or plan for sustainability of the intervention at the conclusion of the project. While outcome scores were lower for systems redesign and patient care projects (i.e., the aims were harder to meet on more ambitious projects), those projects had a greater potential for lasting impact. Some student projects rose to the level of sustainable and meaningful change. Examples of each of the types of projects are highlighted (and shared with permission) in Table 9.2.

While scholarship was not included among the course objectives, a fraction of students used their QI projects as a catalyst for scholarship opportunities. Students presented the results of their QI efforts at regional and national conferences, and some were published in peer-reviewed journals.

Faculty Project Sponsor Survey

We invited faculty project sponsors over the past two academic years (2017–2018 and 2018–2019, n = 53) to participate in an anonymous 7-question survey online about their experience with being a sponsor. Twenty-two faculty responded (response rate 41.5%). The results revealed that 81% of sponsors were somewhat or very comfortable with their QI skills prior to working as a QI sponsor. There was no significant change in the level of their QI skills as a result of participating as a sponsor for a student QI project. Most sponsors (72%) spent, on average, 21 to 40 hours mentoring the student over a 3-month period, while others spent more

than 40 hours. None spent less than 20 hours. Overall, 95% of the faculty surveyed would recommend being a sponsor to a colleague. When asked about the impact that student QI projects had on patient care or clinical processes, faculty unanimously agreed that student-driven QI projects improved patient care or processes in small ways.

Evidence for Institutional, Community, and Patient Care Impact

Admittedly, a program such as ours that was designed with student learning as the primary aim does not simultaneously aspire to make significant impacts on the institution or community. The nature of the projects being small scale and student run inevitably results in most projects having marginal impact on the institution or community. We recognize that this program was not designed to align the needs of the institution, community, or patient care with the student QI projects. Thus, the larger or longer-term impacts are minimal and harder to measure, let alone to determine causality.

However, some students choose to complete their projects in Vanderbilt's student-run free clinic, called Shade Tree Clinic. Students often gravitate toward this option because it is a familiar clinical setting and one in which they have control over the environment and systems processes. The impact of continuously supporting multiple QI projects at a single clinical site has resulted in a culture of improvement where QI projects often flourish. Dr. Robert Miller, the Shade Tree Clinic co-medical director, commented about the impact of students as change agents:

Most US medical schools have created student-run community clinics. The medical services vary in services and scope of care, but all provide opportunities for learning, which do not exist in standard medical school curriculums. Students working in these clinics have the opportunity to observe specific barriers to health care. They identify issues which may enhance or detract from optimal care. The result is that the students take ownership of their clinics and improve the system of care. My observation in our institution is that medical students take ownership of their clinic services and regularly offer ideas and solutions to enhance care. Their perspectives not only help the clinic that they run but are frequently transferred to their parent institutions to improve care. Medical students represent a tremendous (untapped) source of quality improvement.

Using a programmatic evaluation framework, we presented evidence of effectiveness related to the learner reaction and perceived value. In general, students are pleased with the ability to find a project that is meaningful for them

TABLE 9.2 Examples of Student-Led Quality Improvement Projects

Patient Education Example

Project title: Preoperative Education to Reduce Sinus Surgery Postoperative Callbacks

Clinical site: Otolaryngology (ENT)

Problem statement: Perioperative education plays an important role in patient outcome and satisfaction. Two studies have looked at perioperative counseling for colorectal surgery and found that patient education results in shorter length of stay for patients.

Aim statement: Our goal is to reduce average endoscopic sinus surgery 2-week postoperative call rate by at least 20%, from 0.56 to 0.45 in the Vanderbilt University Medical Center (VUMC) otolaryngology clinic by the end of April 2019.

Intervention: For Plan-Do-Study-Act (PDSA) cycle 1, we utilized a preoperative phone call script to contact patients undergoing endoscopic sinus surgery at VUMC 5–10 days prior to their operation. This script focused on topics that were frequently asked in the postoperative period as determined by our Pareto diagram. The number of completed calls and time spent on these calls was recorded. We then followed these patients and documented the number of postoperative calls in a 2-week period. For PDSA 2, we reviewed the topics of the postoperative calls and revised our script to more adequately address those topics and shortened the script to ease patient understanding.

Outcome(s): Our data shows that we achieved a median postoperative callback rate of 0.45 with our two PSDA cycles. We completed preoperative phone calls to 20 patients, with each week ranging from 1 to 5 patients contacted. We are successful in reaching our goal of a 20% reduction in the median postoperative callback rate.

Provider Education Example

Project title: Decreasing the Rate of Incorrectly Placed Radiology Orders: A Quality Improvement Project

Clinical site: Orthopedics outpatient clinic

Problem statement: Radiographic imaging of the musculoskeletal system is essential to the practice of orthopedic surgery. Errors in radiology (i.e., errors of laterality, incorrect views) can result in excessive radiation exposure, delays in diagnosis, and unnecessary surgical interventions, among other complications.

Aim statement: By the end of October 2018, we will reduce the rate of incorrectly placed radiology orders in Vanderbilt outpatient orthopedic clinics from an average of 11.2 per month to 7 or less per month by focusing on improving errors of laterality.

Intervention: Created a document throughout clinic (e.g., at workstations, near computers), reminding nurses to check laterality when placing radiology orders.

Outcome(s): The rate of incorrectly placed orders per month decreased from 11.2 to 6.3 following the first PDSA cycle, and there was a shift in the run chart from April 2018 to September 2018.

System Redesign Example

Project title: Vanderbilt Children's Cath Lab Efficiency Initiative

Clinical site: Vanderbilt Children's Hospital (VCH) catheterization lab

Problem statement: Operating Room (OR) inefficiency is a problem for academic medical centers and most initiatives to improve OR efficiency have not shown sustained results after team training or leadership changes.

Aim statement: Reduce the total time between VCH pediatric catheterization cases by 10% (44–39.6 min) by July 2019 (1 year).

Intervention: Initiated staffing improvements, including increasing nurse shift from 8 to 10 hours, instituted a nurse practitioner (NP) to aid with discharge from the post-anesthesia care unit (PACU), using research staff to enter data, and improved scheduling of catheterization procedures.

Outcome(s): Turnaround time (TAT) and first case start (FCS) both improved by at least 10%, which may reflect a combination of improved team problem awareness and communication, as well as staffing and technological improvements. The VCH catherization lab was also awarded a third room due to their improvement efforts.

Continued

TABLE 9.2 Examples of Student-Led Quality Improvement Projects—cont'd	
Patient Care Example *Project title:* De-Implementation of Empiric Vancomycin Use in Clinically Stable Urology Inpatients *Clinical site:* Urology inpatient	*Problem statement:* Vancomycin and zosyn are commonly used empiric antibiotics in the hospital when an infection is suspected. However, with higher doses and longer duration of vancomycin use, the risk of nephrotoxicity increases. Furthermore, the combination of vancomycin and zosyn carries an increased risk for acute kidney injury. *Aim statement:* Our goal is to reduce the rate of empiric IV vancomycin use among clinically stable urology inpatients by 50% from a baseline average of 191 days of therapy/1000 patient days (DOT/1000d) to an average of 95 DOT/1000d by the end of April 2019. *Intervention:* PDSA cycle 1 included developing a vancomycin de-implementation protocol, presenting this evidence-based protocol to the Urology Department at Grand Rounds, and display the protocol in work areas. PDSA cycle 2 involved encouraging use of the protocol by sending monthly updates of the progress along with email reminders of the protocol and creating visual aids of monthly progress to share with the department. *Outcome(s):* The aim of this project is to reduce inappropriate use of empiric vancomycin in stable surgical inpatients. We met our aim to reduce days of vancomycin therapy by 50% and were able to reduce by 85% from average 191 to 29 DOT/1000d.

and appreciate working together in pairs. Experiencing QI firsthand not only teaches critical systems skills but is also valuable to students' learning and future career. An analysis of the QI projects demonstrates measures of student learning and provides examples of four types of interventions: patient education, provider education, systems redesign, and patient care. Through these types of QI interventions, students act as change agents to add value to the institution and improve care delivery in small, albeit measurable, ways.

RESOURCES NEEDED

The FHD QI courses are supported by a variety of faculty and staff as well as other resources and institutional assets. First and foremost, having strong institutional support and buy-in from leadership is a key component to any successful program, but especially one that requires significant financial support and curricular time.

Vanderbilt University School of Medicine is fortunate to have an affiliation not only with Vanderbilt University Medical Center but also with the Tennessee Valley Health Care system's Nashville Veterans Affairs Hospital. Both institutions have a long history and tradition of excellence in quality and dedication to training individuals with QI skills. This creates a supportive atmosphere wherein many of the faculty at our institution are familiar with or have obtained additional training or certification in QI methods.

That pool of trained faculty allows the FHD course to easily draw on local expertise.

The FHD longitudinal program is administered with the direction of faculty co-course directors. Their primary responsibility is to run the entire FHD series of courses across all years and provide administrative direction and oversight to the program. The faculty block directors are responsible for administering the month-long courses, including teaching, providing feedback, holding weekly office hours, and submitting course grades. The FHD program manager and coordinators assist with all administrative needs. Table 9.3 summarizes the faculty and staff effort required for the FHD QI courses.

In addition to the faculty and staff effort, the QI courses require technology for asynchronous learning, including an online learning management system in which project-related assignments are submitted for feedback.

Students have one half-day of protected time each week (20 hours per month) to complete these course requirements during months they are enrolled in a QI course. During that time, students can work independently on their project or meet with block directors during office hours to get individualized feedback and advice. Classroom space requirements for the course are minimal due to the focus on independent work; however, a single classroom is reserved every Tuesday afternoon to accommodate face-to-face sessions with the students enrolled in each QI course (on weeks 1 and 4) and office hours (on weeks 2 and 3)

TABLE 9.3	Faculty and Staff Effort		
Title	**Number of Individuals**	**Effort (FTE = full-time effort)**	**Roles**
FHD Co-Course Directors	3	0.4 FTE faculty each (1.2 FTE total)	• Provide administrative and educational oversight for the QI courses • Direct course improvement efforts • Manage student- or course-related concerns
QI Course Block Directors	2	0.2 FTE faculty each (or equivalent 0.5 FTE staff effort)	• Provide QI expertise • Administer each of the 3 QI courses monthly • Provide feedback to students on project-related assignments • Respond to student needs • Hold office hours weekly • Issue final grades
Faculty Project Sponsors	Variable, 1 per student project	Volunteer	• Provide clinical microsystem expertise • Assist students with project planning and execution (i.e., identifying a quality gap, collecting baseline data measurement, data access, stakeholder engagement)
FHD Program Manager	1	Full-time	• Lead the administrative team and delegate tasks among the administrative team • Manage course administration tasks, including course improvements • Manage FHD email inbox
FHD Program Coordinator	2	Full-time	• Course build-out and management within the learning management system • Assist with course material distribution, scheduling of classrooms, managing course calendars, other administrative needs

FHD, The Foundations of Healthcare Delivery; *QI*, quality improvement.

with the faculty block directors. In response to scheduling changes prompted by the COVID-19 pandemic, faculty started offering virtual office hours each Tuesday afternoon.

IMPLEMENTATION HISTORY AND STRATEGIES EMPLOYED

We have made innumerable iterations and revisions to the FHD courses in response to student feedback and course evaluations. Importantly, we designed the FHD QI courses during a curricular revision with clear institutional support and buy-in. Even from its inception, our institutional priority was to create a course in which students could take on value-added roles, including being actively engaged in the QI process. The vision was a program in which QI was not an add-on but rather an integral part of the educational experience of the doctor of medicine (MD) degree. This clear directive facilitated the curriculum development

process and allowed us to implement a course that was not only required of all students but was purposefully integrated with other courses. One advantage of developing this longitudinal course during an institution-wide curricular change was that it facilitated an open negotiation about critical curricular time and integration within the third-year schedule.

Another key question during the initial phases of curriculum development was which curricular year was most ideal for fostering QI work. The initial thought was to conveniently use the first-year continuity clinic sites as ideal laboratories for QI work. However, after a pilot, it became obvious to course directors that first-year students did not have the clinical context, comfort level, or professional identity formation required to critically evaluate the clinical practice, identify a problem, and effectively engage in QI work. Second- and fourth-year curricula were less ideal because of other demands, including core clinical clerkships and residency interviews/graduation, respectively.

In our case, the third year was optimal for QI work given that, by then, students have acquired necessary clinical knowledge and context and are ideally prepared and motivated to complete a QI project.

Although QI is a graduation requirement at Vanderbilt, we had to adapt to meet the needs of a variety of unique student cohorts, including dual-degree students and students who complete year-long extracurricular programs (i.e., research). In response to these cohorts, we created two alternative pathways for completing the QI requirement. The QI Advanced Track (QI-AT) is an independent QI pathway for students with previous QI experience or an ongoing project who did not require additional mentorship. Interested students submit an initial application for the QI-AT to FHD course directors that includes a plan for their project and must receive approval prior to beginning. Following the initial approval process, students then proceed to complete the project independently using proscribed project guidelines. Once the project is completed, students can apply for QI-AT credit at which time their project is submitted and graded with the same grading rubrics used in the traditional QI courses. A similar alternative path accommodates the specific needs of MD-PhD dual-degree students in the Medical Scientist Training Program (MSTP). These students complete a modified QI curriculum during their graduate school years that combines the IHI Model for Improvement concepts with the physician-scientist goals of preparation on rigor and reproducibility (RR). Students complete a lab-based QI/RR project with some guidance from FHD course directors and the MSTP that helps them achieve competency in QI concepts by improving a protocol or process in their laboratory environment.

Based on student feedback, we developed and automated a process to gather information about completed student QI projects to act as a clearinghouse of project ideas for students to peruse. This list is updated quarterly and published on our internal course website. This process connects students seeking project ideas to clinical sites or faculty sponsors that have worked with students before on QI projects and identifies past projects that potentially could be continued with additional improvement cycles.

Another important change in recent years was the shift from a pass-fail grading system to the honors/high pass/pass/fail grading system. Using detailed grading rubrics within each course, we had adequate assessment data from student project-related assignments to differentiate high performers from lower performers over the 3-month-long courses. Making this switch and clearly outlining the expectations for an honors project increased the overall rigor and quality of the projects.

KEY ADVICE FOR FEASIBILITY AND SUSTAINABILITY

We have learned many lessons regarding feasibility and sustainability. Listed in this section are the key points of advice for institutions considering a similar program but concerned about whether a program of this scale is feasible or generalizable.

1. *Secure institutional support and stakeholder buy-in.* Find individuals at your institution eager to champion QI work among students—you will need their support to build a successful program. It is hoped that this chapter has provided you with some of the evidence to justify your argument that students as change agents can and do add value to the clinical enterprise by partnering with faculty sponsors in their improvement efforts.

2. *Consider carefully the ideal placement of QI work within the overall degree program.* You need to consider timing with competing demands, the amount of curricular time allotment required, and student preparedness for engaging in QI work. While we have found that QI work is ideal in the third year of medical school after a second year of core clinical clerkships, many institutions will have differing curricular structures and may find that students are primed at a slightly different timeframe.

3. *Engage and pay dedicated faculty to oversee projects.* Paying for faculty effort is important to providing feedback that guides students' projects. Available time on a weekly basis to dedicate to students is more important than QI expertise, since training resources and programs are readily available for interested faculty to quickly learn the content. Paying these individuals is key to a successful program; however, some cost-saving measures could be used in resource-limited scenarios. For example, we have successfully used a staff member with QI expertise in lieu of a faculty member, which saved on some costs considering the differential in pay between staff and faculty when factoring for full-time effort. Another option, which we have not used, is a fixed lump sum payment.

4. *Provide students adequate and timely feedback.* The importance of this cannot be overstated. The process and timeliness of faculty feedback to students has been a key driver of improvement efforts for the program. Students continue to crave timely guidance and feedback in order to effectively incorporate feedback into their project in real time.

5. *Seek out faculty project sponsors who volunteer to support student-driven projects.* These individuals need not be paid to be satisfied with their experience; offering nonmonetary incentives (e.g., Maintenance of Certification

credit, participation awards or certificates, opportunities for scholarship that assist with promotion or tenure) can help keep this group engaged year after year.

6. *Advise students to seek feasible projects.* Having a list of past projects available for students can help them get a sense for what others have done in the past and connect them with willing and eager mentors and clinical settings. Directing students to clinical sites, such as student-run clinics, where they have optimal control over the processes and access to clinical data can be a beneficial way to promote autonomy and avoid common pitfalls in change management.

7. *Adapt curriculum to meet the needs and resources of your institution.* We have successfully employed modifications to the curriculum as described in the examples of alternative pathways. These examples prove that adaptations to the outlined curricular structure also meet the course goals using a different approach or shorter time frame. Such adaptations provide a template for institutions with limited curricular time or course support that are nonetheless interested in starting a QI curriculum but may not be able to do so in the same format.

8. *Take the first step and do not forget to employ a QI process to your curriculum.* As faculty interested in QI processes, it is imperative that we apply the same principles to our work as educators. With the help of rapid-cycle feedback and course evaluation data, we have iteratively improved the course year by year. The course structure and data described here are a result of years of curricular improvement intended to refine the curriculum to meet the needs of students and the institution. We make no assumptions that we have gotten it "right" and that the structure and course will not change again. We take the QI process seriously and will continue to refine it. That said, you should take heart in knowing that any step forward is a step in the right direction and through employing a mindset of continuous improvement, you too can move your institution closer to building a vision of students becoming change agents.

CONCLUSION

The Foundations of Healthcare Delivery (FHD) Quality Improvement (QI) courses at Vanderbilt University Medical School seek to involve students as change agents in small tests of change in a clinical learning environment with which they are familiar. Our course prioritizes teaching the process and maximizing student autonomy over meeting institutional or faculty needs. Throughout the QI courses, students not only learn fundamental improvement concepts—they are also asked to implement changes. In general, students enjoy the opportunity to learn QI principles

and feel that this is important to their future careers. Our experience is that timing within the curriculum is an important consideration. In order to ensure success, students require guidance in the form of mentorship in the clinical learning environment and timely faculty feedback. Students should be directed to projects that are small in scope and ideally in a setting with which they are familiar. This allows students access to data sources and often results in increased autonomy over the change process, all of which increases learner satisfaction and facilitates learning. An analysis of student-led QI projects reveals that student projects fell into four categories: patient education, provider education, system redesign, and patient care. While patient or provider education projects tended to be lower impact, the outcomes were easy to achieve. On the other hand, system redesign and patient care projects were more ambitious and harder to achieve but had a higher potential for lasting impact. In summary, when students are given the opportunity to engage in QI projects of their choosing, they learn the process of improvement and step into the role of change agent within the clinical environment. While not all student projects are of equal value to the system, in this curricular model *all* learners come away with the knowledge of how to evaluate, plan, and implement changes. The hope is that by nurturing future change agents, we are preparing a new generation of medical graduates with skills to tackle increasingly complex challenges throughout their careers.

STUDENT REFLECTIONS

At Vanderbilt, we enter our quality improvement coursework with clerkships and 2 years of health systems science under our belts. Because of this, we get to approach our quality improvement (QI) projects with context for the work and familiarity with systems thinking. My project arose organically from idiosyncrasies that I noticed as a clerkship student, and previous coursework gave me an interprofessional lens that proved critical for a pediatric emergency department (ED) project. The QI curriculum prompted me to physically go to the ED and talk with the stakeholders, where I learned I was completely wrong about the problem's root. Instead of taking a hierarchical approach, the QI framework led me to seek understanding. The most important question turned out to be "what do our nurses need?" Shifting my understanding of the problem helped me approach the intervention constructively, but I think ultimately it will make me a stronger resident and physician with the skills to ask careful and integrative questions.

> *Whereas large systems issues might otherwise be overwhelming, I find the QI framework quite hopeful—I think it's a very accessible action plan for the optimistic realist. As an aspiring emergency medicine resident, I will undoubtedly encounter challenging outcomes of imperfect systems, so having this toolset to address those challenges offers me a greater sense of agency, curiosity, and confidence that meaningful change is possible. I think QI in general narrows the gap between the values that make medicine such a satisfying career and the systems dilemmas that challenge us.*
>
> **—Catherine Havemann, MD candidate,**
> *Vanderbilt University Medical School Class of 2021*

REFERENCES

1. Miller BM, Moore DE, Stead WW, Balser JR. Beyond Flexner: a new model for continuous learning in the health professions. *Acad Med.* 2010;85(2):266–272.
2. Skochelak SE, Stack SJ. Creating the Medical Schools of the Future. *Acad Med.* 2017;92(1):16–19.
3. Skochelak SE, Hammoud MM, Lomis KD, et al. In: Skochelak SE, ed. *Health Systems Science.* 2nd ed. Philadelphia: Elsevier; 2020.
4. Gonzalo JD, Dekhtyar M, Starr SR, et al. Health systems science curricula in undergraduate medical education: identifying and defining a potential curricular framework. *Acad Med.* 2017;92(1):12–131.
5. Corrigan JM, Donaldson MS, Kohn LT, Maguire SK. *Crossing the Quality Chasm: A New Health System for the 21st Century.* Washington, DC: Institute of Medicine; 2001.
6. Kohn LT, Corrigan JM, Donaldson MS. *To Err Is Human. Building a Safer Health System.* Washington, DC: Committee on Quality of Health Care in America, Institute of Medicine; 1999.
7. National Academies of Medicine. *Health Professions Education: A Bridge to Quality.* April 18, 2003. http://www.nationalacademies.org/hmd/Reports/2003/Health-Professions-Education-A-Bridge-to-Quality.aspx. Accessed January 5, 2021.
8. Nelson EP, Batalden PB, Godfrey MM, Lazar JS. *Value by Design: Developing Clinical Microsystems to Achieve Organizational Excellence.* Hoboken, NJ: John Wiley & Sons; 2011.
9. Dornan T, Boshuizen H, King N, Scherpbier A. Experience-based learning: a model linking the processes and outcomes of medical students' workplace learning. *Med Educ.* 2007;41(1):84–91.
10. Institute for Healthcare Improvement (IHI) Open School. http://www.ihi.org/education/IHIOpenSchool/Pages/default.aspx. Accessed January 5, 2021.
11. Frank JR, Snell LS, ten Cate O, Holmboe ES. Competency-based medical education: theory to practice. *Med Teach.* 2010;32(8):638.
12. Frye AW, Hemmer PA. Program evaluation models and related theories: AMEE guide no. 67. *Med Teach.* 2012;34(5):e288–e299.
13. Kirkpatrick D. Revisiting Kirkpatrick's four-level-model. *Train Develop.* 1996;1:54–59.

10

Community Health in Action: The A.T. Still University's School of Osteopathic Medicine in Arizona

Joy H. Lewis and Kate Whelihan

LEARNING OBJECTIVES

1. Define the elements of community-oriented primary care (COPC).
2. Discuss strategies for engaging students and community organizations in COPC projects.
3. Describe the steps involved in implementing and evaluating student COPC projects.
4. Explore the COPC toolkit.
5. Describe examples of successful student-led COPC projects.

OUTLINE

CHAPTER SUMMARY

In this chapter, we briefly describe our unique community health center–based distributed model of undergraduate medical education while we focus on our approach to teaching students about community-oriented primary care (COPC) and our requirement that student teams conduct COPC projects during their second year of undergraduate medical education. COPC is taught as a framework for delivery that plays a special role in meeting the needs of communities in the evolving landscape of health care. These yearlong projects are designed to address issues local leaders, community members, and medical students consider important. The student-directed projects add value for patients, health centers, and communities. We describe methods and tools to implement and evaluate student-led COPC projects.

INTRODUCTION

In 2007, A.T. Still University established its second osteopathic medical school, the School of Osteopathic Medicine in Arizona (ATSU-SOMA), with an innovative curricular model based on a unique partnership with the National Association of Community Health Centers (NACHC). This model utilizes a total immersion-training approach in which students are embedded in **community health centers** (CHCs) for years 2 to 4 of their undergraduate medical education (UME). ATSU-SOMA fulfilled a national need for an innovative medical education program to prepare physicians for the unique demands of working in America's CHCs—the safety net for nearly 30 million patients regardless of ability to pay.[1,2]

Through our relationship with NACHC, ATSU-SOMA formed partnerships with member CHCs across the US, from New York to Hawaii. These CHC partners serve as community campuses that offer students contextual learning environments. The community campuses and locations have evolved and changed over the years. The community partner sites as of September 2020 are listed in Table 10.1. This distributed, contextual model with early clinical training experiences affords students opportunities to become part of the CHC system and to study the social, economic, and medical needs of patients and communities. Students spend their first year of UME together as a class on our Mesa, Arizona campus. They then spend years 2 to 4 living, studying, and working in their new CHC communities. Students are distributed in groups of approximately 10, and all students are assigned to their designated community partner site prior to matriculation. ATSU-SOMA's unique model employs a variety of curricular innovations to implement a fully accredited, decentralized curriculum. Embedding students within care delivery systems enables improved continuity of care, development of employment bonds, and deeply rooted local connections. By working and living in these settings, ATSU-SOMA students develop an authentic perspective regarding the challenges patients experience when trying to access care (e.g., financial, linguistic, cultural, geographic, mobility related, etc.). Thus, they learn how to actively contribute to improving the health outcomes of vulnerable individuals and populations. To further this aim and to gain understanding of methods to assess and improve population health, all students participate in a yearlong course sequence in epidemiology, biostatistics, and preventive medicine. Students develop, implement, and evaluate **community-oriented primary care** (COPC) projects during these courses. Students work with CHC leaders, community members, and others to develop and implement projects that address important **social determinants of health** (SDOH).

ATSU-SOMA students usually have strong community service backgrounds and an expressed interest in serving the underserved. These traits are sought in the recruitment process and heavily considered for enrollment. ATSU-SOMA strives to build on these inherent characteristics by instilling within students the compassion, experience, knowledge, and skills required to address the whole person and shape health care in communities where needs are greatest.

During the second year of UME, students transition to their community partner sites. Through lectures, small-group activities, and experiential learning, students are thoroughly immersed in the local health system and gain an understanding of community health practices. Each community site is led by two physician educators who serve as regional directors of medical education (RDMEs). The site is also staffed by a regional education coordinator. Each RDME team conducts a week-long orientation for incoming second-year students. During this time, students meet with leaders from their health center, engage with CHC staff and clinicians, and learn more about the communities they are joining. Each orientation program covers the logistics

| TABLE 10.1 ATSU-SOMA Community Partner Sites as of September 2020 |||
Organization Name	City	State
Waianae Coast Comprehensive Health Center	Waianae	Hawaii
HealthPoint	Renton	Washington
Northwest Regional Primary Care Association	Portland	Oregon
Family Healthcare Network	Visalia	California
San Ysidro Health Center	San Ysidro	California
North Country Healthcare	Flagstaff	Arizona
Adelante Healthcare	Phoenix	Arizona
El Rio Community Health Center	Tucson	Arizona
Community Healthcare Clinic of Wichita Falls	Wichita Falls	Texas
Southern Illinois Healthcare Foundation	Centreville	Illinois
Near North Health Service Corporation	Chicago	Illinois
HealthSource	Mt. Orab	Ohio
Beaufort-Jasper-Hampton Comprehensive Health Services	Ridgeland	South Carolina
The Wright Center	Scranton	Pennsylvania
Sunset Park Family Health Center	Brooklyn	New York

required for distance education and for navigating the local CHC and health care system. In addition, the RDMEs and other staff provide in-depth explorations that cover the history, unique needs, and some important aspects of each community. While each orientation is unique, all focus on developing respect, understanding, and appreciation for the various cultures and people in the communities that the students are joining.

For example, many students who join the Beaufort Jasper Hampton Comprehensive Health Services (BJHCHS) community—based in Ridgeland, South Carolina—are not from the area and are not familiar with the Lowcountry of South Carolina. Their RDMEs give them an introduction to the people and places so that students understand from day one who they are working with and taking care of.

RDMEs introduce the students to the senior staff and the physicians they will be working with. They take the students to all 9 of their sites, a tour that spans over 200 miles round trip. This tour is a way to ensure that every staff member of the BJHCHS meets the students and knows they are part of their health center. The RDMEs also take the students to the Penn Center, the first school for freed slaves in the southern US.[3] It was established in 1862 by Quaker and Unitarian missionaries and is now a cultural and educational center. The center is an important part of the history of the area, showing the juxtaposition of the African American and Gullah-Geechie communities who have influenced many aspects of local culture. RDMEs also take the students to the camps where migrant farmworkers live and work. These camps are home to part of the population served by BJHCHS; it is important for students to experience where these community members live and work.

Students who join the Waianae Coast Comprehensive Health Center (WCCHC) in Waianae, Hawaii, learn about the history, culture, and needs of native Pacific Islanders. The students meet with community leaders, are introduced to the Hawaiian language, and engage with the practitioners at the WCCHC Native Hawaiian Traditional Healing Center.[4] This center promotes native Hawaiian healing and cultural education, practices, and traditions. Students learn about Lomilomi (Hawaiian massage therapy), Laau Lapaau (herbal medicine), Laau Kahea (spiritual healing), and Hooponopono (conflict resolution) while also gaining a deeper understanding of the history, traditions, and unique strengths of and challenges faced by the community.

Students at our Mt. Orab, Ohio, location are introduced by the HealthSource Community Relations director to the populations served. For example, the students are provided information about vulnerable populations who are at risk for food insecurity. Some students volunteer to prepare food bags that provide recipes and enough ingredients for a meal for a family of four. The students are also introduced

to the Cincinnati Music and Wellness program, which uses recreational music making to work with various populations, such as older refugees.[5] This program also provides civic instruction to help people with their citizenship exams.

Students in Portland, Oregon, are introduced to several different clinics, each with a distinct patient population. Each clinic provides an orientation, and students present case reports from their assigned clinics, sharing information about the various populations with the full student group. For example, one clinic provides a significant amount of gender confirmation services, another serves a large population of people experiencing homelessness, and another provides immigration physicals for the state of Oregon. There, the students use translators for nearly every encounter and have interesting cultural expriences to share with their group.

In Brooklyn, New York, the RDMEs aim to introduce the students to the wide variety of people and cultures served by their health center. The various health center sites serve strikingly distinct populations. It is common at each site to have the majority of patients speak their first language and to have maintained traditions and cultural beliefs from their countries of origin. As a fun way to get to know the people and places where they will be working, the students visit every clinical site and then usually have lunch each day at a local community spot where they are joined by different medical directors. Orientation week has included the Brooklyn Chinatown center (Chinese food), Flatbush center (Carribean food), Sunset Park center (Spanish food), and Park Ridge (Arab cuisine).[6] In addition, students visit Brooklyn landmarks to help them feel at home in their new community. Finally, the students are introduced to the Family Support Services Center,[7] where they get to know the many programs in place supporting food pantries, exercise classes, adult education, early childhood education, workforce development, and more.

These orientation sessions set the stage for the years to come. Students rapidly become part of each community and the contextual learning environments. Early in the development of our program, we looked at community projects as a way that our students could give back to their health centers and the communities they serve. These started off as informal projects, such as contributions to local health fairs or other programs where students would perform a community service. In 2011, we introduced the yearlong course sequence in epidemiology, biostatistics, and preventive medicine (EBPM). In keeping with the mission to train compassionate physicians and health care leaders who serve medically underserved populations with a focus on research and COPC, we formalized the community projects; developed detailed criteria, tools, templates, and rubrics; and incorporated them into the yearlong EBPM course sequence.

Students are taught to design, implement, and evaluate their own COPC projects. Utilizing the framework for COPC outlined by the Institute of Medicine (renamed the National Academy of Medicine in 2015),[8,9] students work with health center leadership and community stakeholders to address important issues and the needs of patients and communities served by the health centers.

DESCRIPTION OF THE COMMUNITY PROJECT PROGRAM AT A.T. STILL UNIVERSITY'S SCHOOL OF OSTEOPATHIC MEDICINE IN ARIZONA

COPC is a model of primary care that stresses the role of community context in individual health. COPC is defined as "a continuous process by which primary health care is provided to a defined community on the basis of its assessed health needs through the planned integration of public health practice with the delivery of primary care services."[10] The aim of COPC is to systematically identify and act on community health needs using public health principles from epidemiology, primary care, and preventive medicine.

COPC is a framework (Fig. 10.1) for health care delivery that serves as the bridge between clinical medicine and public health and is a way for practitioners to address SDOH through community education or other programming. It is an ideal structure for medical students to utilize. The students are able to use their early medical knowledge along with their many other skills, including creativity,

communication, teaching techniques, organizational skills, and many other attributes to develop, implement, and evaluate innovative projects that provide important services and programs for patients, communities, and health centers. Fig. 10.2 defines the elements and process of COPC.

The COPC projects serve as experiential learning opportunities. These allow students to become familiar with community health, research methods, program development, and evaluation. At each CHC campus, students work in teams of 5 to 10 and are encouraged to pursue a project of interest to them that also directly involves and impacts the community.

Although community-based research and program evaluation adhere to different guidelines than more traditional

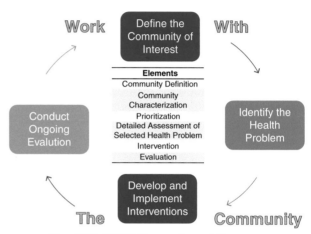
Fig. 10.2 COPC Elements and Process.

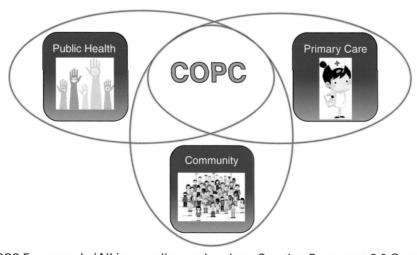
Fig. 10.1 COPC Framework. (All images licensed under a Creative Commons 3.0 Generic License.)

empirical research, students are taught to follow all of the steps required of any investigator. Students conduct needs assessments, perform literature reviews, develop detailed project proposals, and submit their projects for human subjects review. Student teams implement these projects and conduct ongoing evaluations of the process and outcomes. All students complete required trainings in human subjects protection and financial conflict of interest, and all projects are submitted to the ATSU Arizona Institutional Review Board (IRB).

The community project is designed to be developed, implemented, evaluated, and documented within the academic year. The project steps and required assignments are divided between two semesters.

Although a student's project begins at the start of the second year of UME, students are usually introduced to the concept of community projects through a live large-group presentation held at the end of the first year. During this session, course instructors explain the history and importance of the projects, describe the required steps, provide examples of past projects, and address questions. This way, students have some working knowledge of project requirements when they arrive at their new community. They take part in orientation and meet CHC leaders already aware of the COPC framework. In 2020, due to the COVID-19 pandemic and resultant need for distance learning, this orientation was changed to a recorded lecture followed by individual video conference meetings with each CHC team. These meetings occurred early in the orientation week.

Toward the end of orientation week, students start to conduct a formal community needs assessment. They are instructed to obtain data on community demographics, identify existing SDOH, review performance measures from their CHC, and review any other statistics relevant to their interests and the needs of the community. Students are provided detailed needs assessment resources where they can find population-based data and resources related to health equity. Table 10.2 provides examples of these resources.

In addition to finding literature and evaluating data on these areas, each team is required to perform a minimum of three interviews with CHC stakeholders. Interviews are typically conducted with members of CHC leadership, directors of community programs, and CHC patients or program participants. These interviews serve as an opportunity for students to learn firsthand the priorities of the CHC and its patients. The interviews also serve as a way to form connections for collaborative project efforts.

Using the information from the needs assessment and interviews, groups then develop a topic. They submit a topic idea with a brief description of why it is important and a tentative outline of a project plan. The topic is expected to reflect the data collected and the input received while fitting into the COPC framework with a focus on SDOH. We review each topic idea and meet with each student team to help formulate the project proposal. These meetings are intended to ensure that each project has realistic goals/objectives, meets the requirements and time frame of the course, follows the COPC framework, and is supported by the CHC. We may meet with teams multiple times before a topic idea is agreed upon.

Once students receive approval to continue, student groups perform additional background research and create a detailed annotated bibliography. With help from the literature and further discussions with CHC leaders and course directors, students then write their project proposal. The proposal includes the following sections: (1) background, (2) purpose, (3) executive summary, (4) elements considered, (5) project questions, (6) goals and objectives, and (7) methods. In the proposal template, we intentionally do not ask for hypotheses. These projects are not about testing hypotheses; instead, they are meant to produce interventions evaluated by process and outcome measures. We also use the term *project questions* instead of *research questions*. The majority of the projects are not classified as research. Some will be quality improvement; others will be program development and program evaluation. Students are taught sound research methods, and they use appropriate methods for their projects. However, forgoing the term *research* opens up the possibilities and allows the students to emphasize other elements of the work besides quantifiable outcomes.

Student teams cannot implement their projects until the IRB provides approval or designates the project as exempt from IRB oversight. Many of the projects submitted are considered exempt or nonjurisdiction. These are projects that pose less than minimal risk to human subjects and are not considered to be research, as defined by the Codified Federal Regulations, 45 CFR 46 §46.102.[11] Some health centers have their own IRB or research committee. Student teams are responsible for identifying their local health center requirements and must submit applications to the local research oversight committees in addition to the Arizona IRB.

Most student teams receive their IRB determination by the end of semester 1 or start of semester 2. Teams typically then spend 1 to 3 months conducting and evaluating their projects. Students are required to write an abstract summarizing their project and key findings and to create a poster documenting their work. Student teams also create video presentations of their projects to share with the ATSU-SOMA, NACHC, and health center communities. The videos provide an opportunity for the students to express personal stories and to explain why they developed

TABLE 10.2 Examples of Needs Assessment and Healthy Equity Resources

Resource Title	Sponsoring Agency	Contents
Culture of Health Program	National Academy of Medicine	Evidence-based strategies to bring about the transformation necessary to dismantle structural racism and ultimately achieve health equity for all.
Healthcare Innovations Exchange	Agency for Healthcare Research and Quality	Information from projects that have been undertaken to improve health and wellness and to reduce disparities.
State Health Facts	Kaiser Family Foundation	Up-to-date state-level health data categorized by various topics.
Health System Tracker	Peterson Center on Healthcare and Kaiser Family Foundation	Up-to-date information on trends, drivers, and issues that impact the performance of the health care system. Also illustrates how different parts of the system are performing relative to one another.
HealthLandscape	American Academy of Family Physicians and Robert Graham Center	Interactive mapping tool with health data and searchable social determinants of health data repository.
HRSA Data Warehouse	Health Resources and Services Administration (HRSA)	Data, dashboards, maps, reports, locators, APIs, and downloadable data files on HRSA's public health programs.

their project, why they feel it is important, what impact they feel they had, and what they gained from the experience. Table 10.3 provides the toolkit sections, project course assignment deliverables, and the timeline.

The student projects vary greatly, reflecting the different community needs and the various interests and talents of our students. For example, one year, students provided oral health education to elementary school children in rural Ohio. As part of this education program, the ATSU-SOMA students performed and recorded a music video called "White Tooth Bling." The video was set to a popular song and showcased the students' creativity, musical abilities, and videography skills. In Chicago, students created a mindfulness and meditation DVD in which they performed the music, song, and spoken word. They studied the perceived benefit of guided mindfulness and meditation exercises for persons experiencing homelessness and for other vulnerable populations.

Our most sustained project was established in 2012 at our Waianae, Hawaii campus.[12] That year, students started a program they called Mini-Docs. Through partnership with a local elementary school, ATSU-SOMA students created and delivered lessons to third grade students on health topics. Each week, the elementary students were encouraged to share what they learned with their family and friends. To document this shared learning, the elementary students brought a form home and asked their parent or caregiver to write down a sentence or two about what they learned from their child. One of the early forms filled out by an elementary student's father stated "I learned to control my anger, to not have a heart attack." At the conclusion of the program, the elementary students were graduated as "miniature doctors" who could play a role in improving community health knowledge.

The Mini-Doc health education program was designed to be reproducible in an effort to combat the prevalence of preventable chronic diseases. We also hoped to spark an interest in health care careers to create a pipeline of future community health center physicians and other health professionals. Student teams in Hawaii have continued the Mini-Doc tradition with various schools and in partnership with nursing education programs and other community organizations. Each ATSU-SOMA team makes the project their own and addresses current issues in innovative ways. The most recent student team introduced education related to mental health disorders to destigmatize depression and other mental health issues. The team also introduced substance misuse education. One interesting side note, a teacher from the first school where our UME students implemented the Mini-Doc program was inspired by our students and their public health education program. She tells us that her work with our students led her to seek further education in public health and health administration. She is now a community health center executive working in Hawaii.

Student projects can build off of prior year projects at one location or be informed by past projects at any location. In 2012 to 2013, students in Portland, Oregon, identified

TABLE 10.3	Toolkit Sections, Project Assignments, and Timeline		
Sections	**Contents**	**Corresponding Assignments**	**Associated Timeline**

Introduction	Statement on Academic Integrity
	How to Use the Toolkit
	Assignment Due Dates
	Introduction to COPC
		Sign attestation stating
		    reviewed syllabus and
		    reviewed requirements
			Start of Month 1
			    (Late August)

Project Preparation	Preparing for Your Project
	Needs Assessment Resources
	Conducting a Literature Search
		CHC Needs Assessment and
		    Topic Development
			End of Month 1
			    (Late September)

Project Proposal	Instructions Guide to Using Proposal Template Grading Rubric	Project Proposal	End of Month 2 (Late October)
IRB Application	Introduction to IRB IRB Application Tips Grading Rubric	IRB Application	Month 3 (Mid-to-late November)
Project Completion	Instructions—Abstract/Poster/Video Grading Rubrics Resources on How to Make a Poster	Project Abstract	Month 7 (Mid- March)
		Project Poster	Start of Month 9 (Early May)
		Video Presentation	Start of Month 9 (Early May)

the problem of opiate overdose among IV heroin users as a preventable cause of death impacting the community around them. The students developed a relationship with the Clark County Public Health department and their harm reduction/needle exchange program.[13,14] The students intended to provide community-based training to increase access to naloxone in the community. By the end of the academic year, the students had succeeded in securing the required relationships between the organizations and the independent IRBs needed to work together. Unfortunately, the partnerships and agreements took too long to develop, preventing this cohort of students from implementing their program.

The student team documented their efforts and their belief that a low-cost overdose training program could be adopted with an established needle exchange program. They asserted that this project could be offered or implemented in facilities located where an intravenous drug use community exists. Their beliefs were well founded. At the beginning of the 2013 to 2014 academic year, the subsequent group of students continued this work with the harm reduction center. These students provided community-based training related to overdose identification, appropriate response, and naloxone use. The training was in conjunction with the distribution of naloxone home kits and covered important information such as the

Good Samaritan Law to improve participants' knowledge and comfort level related to overdose response and naloxone use.

By the time our students presented their project at a national meeting in late August 2014, they had already been notified of 10 overdose reversals performed by people whom they had trained. Both teams of students were informed of these reversals, and all contributed to this outcome.

STUDENT REFLECTION

So far, 10 overdoses have been reversed. I had the chance to speak with one of the participants who used their kit to save a life. He said that if it weren't for the kit, his girlfriend would have died—it took first responders 20 minutes to arrive. Opiate addiction and overdose are a public health crisis. Effects of overdose stem beyond the health care system and can have lasting effects on the community. Community health centers, with their focus on the overall well-being of the local population at large, are uniquely staged to administer a multifaceted naloxone intervention program.

—**Student participant**

Other student groups have built on projects from different CHC sites. Students at one health center identified discrepancies in electronic health record (EHR) documentation when they tried to implement a project to improve colorectal cancer screening in 2014.[15] While this team was not able to increase screening at their health center, they were able to publish their findings to inform others of these documentation discrepancies. The EHR issue they identified was found to be present at other partner health centers, and future student teams at different health centers were able to implement changes and improve colorectal cancer screening documentation and Uniform Data System reporting. Additional examples of projects from 2015 to 2020 are provided in Table 10.4.

While students develop and implement the projects, we provide significant guidance and support along the way. We

TABLE 10.4   Example Projects From 2015 to 2020

Year	CHC Location	Project	Project Description
2015	Flagstaff, AZ	North Country Healthcare Health Partners Program: evaluate patient and provider perceptions	Created health partners program to address social needs by connecting patients to community resources. Students evaluated effectiveness of program by measuring patient satisfaction and success rate for connecting to community resources. Students also evaluated provider views of the program and of the importance of addressing the social determinants of health.
2016	Brooklyn, NY	The effects of a guided education module on awareness and knowledge of contraception among Brooklyn adolescents	Students addressed the high rate of unintended pregnancy among adolescents in Sunset Park (Brooklyn, NY). They provided an internet-based guided education module to adolescents. Medical students assessed knowledge and beliefs before and after completion of the module.
2017	Portland, OR	Resilience training for high school students to reduce the consequences of adversity	Implemented a resilience-building curriculum with high school children who were at high risk for adverse childhood experiences (ACEs). Curriculum included multiple activities addressing values, emotions, positive thinking, reality checks, everyday courage, and role models.
2018	Mt. Orab, OH	Determining the effect of musical therapy and basic hygiene education on improving mental health and well-being of Bhutanese refugees	Refugee populations are often predisposed to mental health disorders due to their difficult transitions and subsequent struggles with cultural identity and changes in family dynamics. Focusing on the Bhutanese refugee population of Cincinnati, students utilized music therapy and preventive care education to address the connection between physical and mental well-being.
2019	Phoenix, AZ	An evaluation of the Nutrition and Health Awareness (NHA) program on health knowledge, health literacy, and activity levels	Students developed the NHA program to educate kids and to cultivate positive attitudes toward health and wellness. Medical students worked with elementary students and implemented a 6-week program with interactive lessons related to exercise, diet, nutrition labels, sugar metabolism, heart disease, and oral hygiene. Children were given accelerometers to measure activity level and for motivation.
2020	Tucson, AZ	Twists, turns, and blockages to colorectal cancer screening follow-up	Contacted health center patients who had Cologuard® screening ordered but had not completed the test. Identified perceived barriers to test completion and provided recommendations to heath center to improve patients' abilities to complete screening.

meet with student teams and RDMEs regularly. We make suggestions, and we know what works and what can be accomplished in the available time frame. The RDMEs are also actively involved with the students, providing guidance, clinical expertise, and knowledge about and connections to the health center and the community.

To assist both students and faculty and to share our methods and materials, we developed a community project toolkit. Toolkit development was supported by the American Medical Association as part of its Accelerating Change in Medical Education Initative. The toolkit contains needs assessment resources, detailed instructions, usable templates, forms, and grading rubrics. Students are encouraged to read through the toolkit and refer to it throughout the year. By following the instructions and consulting the rubrics, student teams can be successful in completing a meaningful project and learning experience.

Learning Goals

Students learn to conduct needs assessments and to analyze and address SDOH for vulnerable populations. In addition, students gain experience in research methods, community-based program development, program implementation, and evaluation. They demonstrate the ability to develop, execute, and evaluate a project, which may be research, quality improvement, or program evaluation. Students develop the ability to create a proposal and an application for the IRB. Students learn to work as part of a team and to work with community-based organizations.

TECHNIQUES TO ASSESS LEARNERS

Each of the project's required assignments are graded based on rubrics provided at the start of the course. The assignments the students turn in for a grade include a community needs assessment; annotated bibliography; project proposal, including a detailed budget; IRB application; project abstract; project poster; and video presentation.

Students are graded as a team on each of their assignment submissions. When grading, greater emphasis is placed on the team's ability to address all sections of the grading rubric and develop a full plan rather than on the robustness of the methodology. It is expected that students will not initially have well-stated project questions, clear goals, and objectives or methods that describe something achievable in the allotted time frame. The focus of the evaluation is on completeness and attention to all components. We then work together to focus the goals and objectives and to outline the specific plans.

It is important to ensure that all project components are aligned; for instance, the stated purpose should match the needs identified and be related to the project questions.

Further, the project questions must be answerable through the proposed methods and the evaluative measures. Historically, students have had difficulty ensuring that all parts of their proposal are aligned. We believe that this is in part due to the students' approach to the group project. Students divide up tasks and different students are assigned to each component. Thus, we may receive beautifully written background information, a clear statement of purpose, well-crafted project questions, important goals and objectives, a well-described implementation plan, and sample evaluation instruments. However, all of these components could be parts of different projects. Over the years, we have learned to emphasize this point and to encourage the students to meet frequently and to share drafts of their work. Teams are also encouraged to have a principal investigator who reviews each section and puts together the document to hand in after reviewing, editing, and ensuring alignment.

In addition to receiving a grade, student teams receive detailed feedback on each assignment. We make it clear that our expectation is that students will incorporate all feedback prior to moving on to the next step in their project development, implementation, or evaluation.

Evaluation Procedures

All ATSU-SOMA courses require students to complete course evaluations. In recent years, the evaluation questions were revised so that each course is assessed the same way. Historically, students were asked to evaluate each course based on unique sets of standards. For the EBPM courses, questions specific to the community projects used to be included. Students were explicitly asked to rate their agreement with the following three statements: *I took an active role in my community project. The project provided me with insights into health-related issues in the community. The project made me feel more connected to my community.* Under the new system, the community project is evaluated as a learning activity and how well it aligned with the course objectives and competencies.

In addition to student evaluations collected at the midpoint and end of each course, an annual review is performed by ATSU-SOMA faculty members of the curriculum committee. The curriculum committee meets with the course director to review the overall performance of the course and discuss recommendations for the following year. This process ensures that the course continues to meet its defined objectives and adheres to the standards established in accordance with the Commission on Osteopathic College Accreditation.

As a supplemental source of evaluation, we keep track of informal feedback received from our fellow faculty, colleagues at NACHC, and our health center partners. At the conclusion of each year, we compile the projects into a sharable format for distribution and welcome discussions and suggestions regarding the work. Although an informal method of evaluation, this feedback often proves most fruitful, as we can gauge the level of interest in topics and spark conversations on sustaining and improving the projects. Additionally, we meet with the chief executive officers of our partner health centers annually, and we review priority areas for research and quality improvement. These meetings help us guide students in their choice of topics to ensure that the topics align with health center priorities.

RESOURCES NEEDED

We describe the implementation of community projects performed as part of our unique program with a distributed model of medical education. The CHC partnerships stem from years of cooperation and collaboration between ATSU, NACHC, and many individual health centers. ATSU-SOMA was founded on this background and was developed explicitly with these partnerships. A team of ATSU and SOMA administrators and faculty work to develop and maintain these relationships. Over the years, new CHC partnerships and new community partner sites have been developed. We utilize a community partner site readiness checklist (Fig. 10.3) to ensure that each new location has adequate leadership support, clinical staff, facilities for student education sessions, relationships with physicians and health systems for clinical rotations, financial resources, and a strong desire to be a community campus for our students. Thus, the implementation of community projects, which include input and cooperation from health center leaders, is possible.

These projects can be implemented by students from more traditionally structured medical education programs. The students require significant supervision and collaboration from advisers and professors, but the projects do not depend on a model in which the education program is distributed or immersed in CHCs. Students can work with local CHCs or other organizations that serve vulnerable populations. Students from any medical education program can work with mentors and can follow the steps outlined for COPC projects. The toolkit can be adapted for any UME or other education program. We have successfully developed COPC project programs within our distributed residency program and have developed a primary care training enhancement fellowship. (Leading and Teaching in the Nation's Health Centers: The Primary Care Transformation Executive Fellowship. September 2018 to August 2023. This program is supported by the Health Resources and Services Administration [HRSA] of the US Department of Health and Human Services [HHS] as part of an award totaling $1,999,650 with 0% financed with nongovernmental sources. The contents of the program are those of the author[s] and do not necessarily represent the official views of, nor an endorsement by, HRSA, HHS, or the US Government.) Our fellows, who are working health center clinicians (MD, DO, or PA) use the methodology we describe and the toolkit to develop, implement, and evaluate COPC projects.

We provide a budget of $600 per project for our students and $1,000 for the fellow project development and implementation. We also provide some financial assistance for travel to present the work. Residency financial support varies by location. Support from the college or university is important whether it is financial or in some other form, such as connections to health center and other community leaders.

DEMONSTRATED VALUE ADDED

The value added by this program can be measured in various ways. Value is added for the students themselves, for health centers and the communities they serve, and for society. Students have described their experiences with the community projects as both rewarding and, at times, frustrating. Many skills are developed and tested through participation in group projects and the unpredictability of real-world program development and evaluation. No matter the topic students pursue, they can benefit from the required learning, teamwork, and community engagement that comprise the community project. The vast majority of students rate their experiences with the projects as favorable. Students have consistently expressed that they understand the value of the community project as a learning experience and as a way of giving back to their CHC community.

> **STUDENT REFLECTION**
>
> The community project has been a really neat opportunity and has pushed me to learn how to do something I've always wanted to do but was intimidated to try, due to my lack of experience.
>
> **—Student participant**

> **STUDENT REFLECTION**
>
> Being immersed in the community health center setting has been an excellent source for information and teaching that I don't believe many others get. Our level of involvement with patients across all spectrums of care has helped me understand how many barriers to health there are and how difficult it can be to navigate the medical system. This experience of true health systems science in action has been invaluable to me.
>
> **—ENS Brysen Keith, MS, SOMA**

A.T.Still Community Partner Site—Readiness Assessment Checklist

Objective
To prepare a checklist of issues for consideration by a community health center (CHC) interested in becoming a community partner site for the A.T. Still University's School of Osteopathic Medicine in Arizona

Background Assumptions
☐ Financially and administratively stable organization with a minimum of 35,000 covered lives, with established CEO and solid quality performance
☐ Experience and track record with health professions education programs or potential faculty who have experience in health education
☐ Affiliation with teaching hospitals and primary care residency programs sufficient to provide clinical rotations for 10 students per year
☐ Commitment to a "grow your own" strategy for training the future CHC workforce
☐ Committed to community oriented primary care

Readiness Assessment
1. Leadership Support
  ☐ CEO, CMO, senior leadership team
  ☐ Board of directors

2. Clinical staff with passion, interest & experience with teaching
  ☐ Potential RDME (Regional Director Medical Education)
  ☐ Motivated potential clinical preceptors

3. Facility "learning space" requirements
  ☐ Conference capacity (seating for 15-30)
  ☐ Quiet environment to allow for student learning with reasonable evening and weekend access
  ☐ Bandwidth for synchronous and asynchronous learning activities and video conferencing
  ☐ IT support

4. Relationship with area clinicians
  ☐ Community teaching hospital(s) which provide services to health center patients and ability to secure required inpatient rotations for third and fourth year students as outlined in the curriculum.
  ☐ Academic medical center(s) /medical school(s)
  ☐ Primary care residency programs (family, internal medicine, pediatrics, ob-gyn)
  ☐ Specialty groups with hospital affiliations (medical, pediatric, ob-gyn, surgery, behavioral health)

5. Financial resources
  ☐ Fiscally sound organization
  ☐ Adequate financial resources to support teaching
  ☐ Willingness and capacity to invest in workforce development

Fig. 10.3 A.T. Still Community Partner Site—Readiness Assessment Checklist.

As a requirement for completion, student teams submit their community project abstracts for consideration to present a poster at the NACHC Community Health Institute and Expo (NACHC CHI). This annual conference, hosted by NACHC, is the largest national gathering of health center stakeholders, employees, and advocates. Conference organizers anticipate the submission of the student abstracts, and a high percentage of ATSU-SOMA student abstracts are accepted each year. During this conference, ATSU-SOMA also hosts an annual education session in which select student teams provide oral presentations on their project experience. All student teams create a project poster regardless of whether or not their project was accepted for presentation at the NACHC meeting. The poster is suitable for presentation at any national meeting. The abstracts, posters, and videos are shared with health center leaders and care teams. These projects and presentations also provide valuable academic scholarly work for clinical faculty.

This opportunity provides a valuable experience for all students to attend a national conference and for many to share their projects with a national audience. Perhaps the most valuable outcome of this conference is the pride and connection that students report feeling. They see the fruition of the valuable contributions they are making to the health center world and the appreciation felt by health center leaders. Students are able to share their innovative projects with other health center workers of all types. In addition to the NACHC CHI, student teams present their work at local, regional, and national conferences. Students have received numerous awards and have gained other positive recognition for their work.

FACULTY REFLECTION

Student community projects have aligned with our ongoing quality innovation projects, underscored our commitment as an FQHC to overcome health care disparities and furthered our footprint of championing the social determinants of health as it relates to the well-being of our community.

—**Douglas J. Spegman, MD,**
Chief Clinical Officer at El Rio Community Health Center

The value added to our partner health centers and the communities they serve is evident from each community project. Much of this benefit is difficult to quantify or prove but can be observed. The projects all include process and outcome evaluations, although the evaluations do not always prove or demonstrate a statistically significant benefit. This is a common issue when doing program evaluation or when conducting research with small populations such as the specific and unique vulnerable populations we work with that are often left out of most large-scale research programs or interventions. Findings from research studies may not apply to these specific groups. The student COPC projects are focused on the specific needs of these groups, and the projects are meant to make a difference but are not designed specifically to prove a statistically significant effect. Our students work with underprivileged and vulnerable children, but our students do not "study" them. Each project includes an evaluation and evidence of benefit, but we do not limit our measure of success to a *p* value. We encourage our students to identify how they made a difference and what can be done in the future to further their work.

When an overdose is reversed by someone trained by our students, the value is evident. When a child learns about nutrition, this knowledge can help her for the rest of her life. When a child learns to embrace exercise, the benefits can occur well beyond our evaluation window. When refugee families are provided education regarding how to obtain health services, are shown a warm welcome, and are made to feel more comfortable engaging with the health system, the benefits can be tremendous. When a student project, or any public health intervention, prevents a negative occurrence, we do not always have a way to measure the benefit. We continue to work to document the value added by these interventions. It is our hope that much of this value is evident by the many projects, the strength of the program, the continued health center support, and the fact that the NACHC continues to showcase our student work to share it with the broader health center community.

The value to the students as health care professionals is also difficult to quantify. We believe that witnessing health care disparities and the plight of vulnerable populations can be emotionally draining for physicians in training and all physicians and other health care professionals.[16,17] Given that our medical interventions affect only a portion of health outcomes and SDOH affect a greater portion,[18] physicians and other health care professionals can feel helpless or frustrated.[19,20] We teach our students to identify and address the SDOH.[21–23] With the COPC program, we give students tools to act and empower them to use their many and varied skills to make a difference in their community. We teach them how to organize their work in this area, how to evaluate it, and how to disseminate it. We believe this can help sustain and empower our students. It is our hope that this work can help protect them from burnout. This protection is unstudied and unproven, but these potential benefits exist and are areas we intend to explore.[24–27]

The value added to society is evident in our graduates' contribution to the workforce. We grow the compassion for the underserved within our students and teach them how to make a difference in the health of the communities they lead. In the real world of caring for our communities, our mission and vision propel graduates to become the next generation of compassionate health care professionals who focus on whole person health care and serve the health care needs of our entire community. Given the extensive training our students receive at their designated community sites and the emphasis our program places on community health, it is not surprising that many of our graduates choose careers in primary care and specialties designated by NACHC as important for the health center movement. Since 2011, ATSU-SOMA has produced an average of 99 graduates annually. Approximately 70% of graduates enter primary care and approximately 89% choose a career in an NACHC-designated needed specialty.

IMPLEMENTATION HISTORY AND STRATEGIES

Since the 2010 to 2011 academic year, students have completed 133 COPC projects. Our UME program expanded in 2019; thus, the 2020 to 2021 academic year will include students at 15 community partner sites. We are encouraging them to pursue projects addressing social justice and health equity. Each year, we evaluate and update aspects of the COPC program in order to keep it current, achievable, and enjoyable. We present students with the current primary care priority areas identified by HRSA and NACHC in addition to the current issues we feel are important.[28]

Since 2012, students have presented a total of 95 posters at the NACHC CHI. In 2013, NACHC started accepting ATSU-SOMA students for a special oral presentation session in addition to the poster presentations. As of September 2019, a total of 45 projects have been presented as part of this session.

KEY ADVICE FOR FEASIBILITY AND SUSTAINABILITY

Students have varying levels of experience and interest in methodology, project development, and program evaluation. It is essential for students to be continually guided by experienced mentors who are available and engaged from project development to project completion. The most successful student teams are supported by invested health center leadership with strong participation from our RDMEs. A dedicated program team is needed for success.

While we instruct students to conduct needs assessments and interviews to help identify areas of need, we also emphasize the importance of finding a topic that is of interest and feels important to them. Working on a project for a full academic year is much easier when it is something you fully believe in. As educators, we have also learned to trust our students. There have been times when students have proposed projects we did not think they would be able to do. They were passionate about their ideas and proved us wrong.

Another major point we stress is that there are many resources available to anyone performing these types of projects. In addition to the tools we developed as part of our COPC toolkit, various databases exist that contain evidence-based programs and validated assessment tools. Students are encouraged to not only be inspired by what they can find in the literature or through existing organizations, they are also encouraged to utilize what they find. Emphasizing this point seems to help with the level of stress. Students do not have to reinvent the wheel. They can use proven programs and strategies, adapt them, and then apply them to their specific community of interest.

REFERENCES

1. Health Resources and Services Adminstration. Health Center Program: Impact and Growth. https://bphc.hrsa.gov/sites/default/files/bphc/about/healthcenterfactsheet.pdf. Updated August 2020. Accessed 06.01.21.
2. National Association of Community Health Centers. America's Health Centers. http://www.nachc.org/wp-content/uploads/2019/09/Americas-Health-Centers-Updated-Sept-2019.pdf. Published August 2019. Accessed 06.01.21.
3. Penn Center. A Timeline of Our History. http://www.penncenter.com/explore-penn-centers-history. Updated 2020. Accessed 06.01.21.
4. Waianae Coast Comprehensive Health Services Center. The Native Hawaiian Traditional Healing Center. http://journey-mobile.wcchc.com/traditional-healing-center.html. Accessed 06.01.21.
5. Cincinatti Music and Wellness Coalition. About Us. https://musicandwellness.net/about. Published 2015. Accessed 06.01.21.
6. NYU Langone Health. Locations. https://nyulangone.org/locations. Updated 2020. Accessed 06.01.21.
7. NYU Langone Health. Community-Based Programs—Family Health Centers at NYU Langone. https://nyulangone.org/locations/family-health-centers-at-nyu-langone/community-based-programs-family-health-centers-at-nyu-langone. Updated 2020. Accessed 06.01.21.
8. Abramson JH, Kark SL. Division of Health Care Services, Institute of Medicine. In: Connor E, Mullan F, eds. *Community Oriented Primary Care: New Directions for Health Services Delivery*. Washington, DC: National Academies Press; 1983.
9. Liaw W, Rankin J, Bazemore A. Module 1: Introduction to community-oriented primary care (COPC). Community Oriented Primary Care Curriculum. https://www.graham-center.org/content/dam/rgc/documents/maps-data-tools/copc-curriculum/COPCModule1-Introduction.pdf. Updated 2020. Accessed 06.01.21.
10. Mullan F, Epstein L. Community-oriented primary care: new relevance in a changing world. *Am J Public Health*. 2002;92(11):1748–1755.
11. Health and Human Services, Office for Human Research Protections. 45 CFR 46. https://www.hhs.gov/ohrp/regulations-and-policy/regulations/45-cfr-46/index.html. Accessed 06.01.21.
12. Waianae Coast Comprehensive Health Center. About Us. https://www.wcchc.com/. Updated 2020. Accessed 06.01.21.
13. Clark County, Washington. Public Health. https://www.clark.wa.gov/public-health. Updated 2020. Accessed 06.01.21.
14. Clark County, Washington. Harm Reduction Syringe Services Program. https://www.clark.wa.gov/public-health/harm-reduction-syringe-services-program. Updated 2020. Accessed 06.01.21.
15. Hill H, Johnson B, Jader L, et al. Quality improvement measures for increasing the colorectal cancer screening rates at a community health center. *JAOA*. 2015;115(12):e20–e24.

16. Ramirez AJ, Graham J, Richards MA, Cull A, Gregory WM. Mental health of hospital consultants: the effects of stress and satisfaction at work. *Lancet*. 1996;347(9003):724–728.

17. Schrijver I. Pathology in the medical profession? Taking the pulse of physician wellness and burnout. *Arch Pathol Lab Med*. 2016;140(9):976–982.

18. Hood CM, Gennuso KP, Swain GR, Catlin BB. County health rankings: relationships between determinant factors and health outcomes. *Am J Prev Med*. 2016;50(2):129–135.

19. Kumar S. Burnout and doctors: prevalence, prevention and intervention. *Healthcare*. 2016;4(3):37.

20. Dyrbye LN, Shanafelt TD, Sinsky CA, et al. Burnout among health care professionals: a call to explore and address this underrecognized threat to safe, high-quality care. Discussion paper: National Academy of Medicine. https://nam.edu/burnout-among-health-care-professionals-a-call-to-explore-and-address-this-underrecognized-threat-to-safe-high-quality-care/. Published July 5, 2017. Accessed 06.01.21.

21. Lewis JH, Whelihan K, Roy D. Teaching students to identify and document social determinants of health. *Adv Med Educ Pract*. 2019;10:653–665.

22. Lewis JH, Whelihan K, Navarro I, Boyle KR. SDH Card Study Implementation Team Community health center provider ability to identify, treat and account for the social determinants of health: a card study. *BMC Fam Prac*. 2016;17(1):121.

23. Lewis JH, Lage OG, Grant BK, et al. Addressing the social determinants of health in undergraduate medical education curricula: a survey report. *Adv Med Educ Pract*. 2020;2020(11):369–377.

24. Linzer M, Visser MR, Oort FJ, et al. Predicting and preventing physician burnout: results from the United States and the Netherlands. *Am J Med*. 2001;111(2):170–175.

25. Cooper CL, Rout U, Faragher B. Mental health, job satisfaction, and job stress among general practitioners. *BMJ*. 1989;298(6670):366–370.

26. Patel UK, Zhang MH, Patel K, et al. Recommended strategies for physician burnout, a well-recognized escalating global crisis among neurologists. *J Clin Neurol*. 2020;16(2):191–201.

27. Odom Walker K, Ryan G, Ramey R, et al. Recruiting and retaining primary care physicians in urban underserved communities: the importance of having a mission to serve. *Am J Public Health*. 2010;100(11):2168–2175.

28. National Assocation of Community Health Centers. Clinical Initiatives. https://www.nachc.org/clinical-matters/current-projects/. Updated 2020. Accessed 06.01.21.

PART III

Implementation

Part III, *Implementation*, examines the nuts and bolts of how to launch and maintain a value-added medical education program. The section utilizes Kern's Curriculum Development Approach and Kotter's Change Management Framework to offer an overarching method for establishing a value-added roles program, from the original idea to the continuing evaluation and feedback of an established enterprise. Chapters span the ongoing cycle of program development, from the initial phase of vision and planning through the maintenance phase of sustaining and growing. The first chapter in this section discusses identifying the problem and establishing a sense of urgency, conducting a needs assessment and gathering a guiding coalition, and developing learning goals along with a shared vision and strategy. The subsequent chapters examine how to communicate the change vision, to empower action and overcome barriers in implementation, to gather short-term wins, to consolidate gains and initiate feedback and evaluation, and to continue evaluation and feedback while anchoring culture change.

11

Envisioning and Planning Value-Added Roles

Suzanne Minor, Gregory W. Schneider, and Jed D. Gonzalo

LEARNING OBJECTIVES

1. Review the evolving concept of a three-pillar medical education model.
2. Summarize Kotter's eight-stage change model.
3. Summarize Kern's six-step approach to curriculum development.
4. Apply Kotter's process and Kern's approach toward planning a medical education curriculum in which students learn experientially through value-added roles.

OUTLINE

CHAPTER SUMMARY

The emerging three-pillar framework of an undergraduate medical education in which health systems science (HSS) is allied with basic science and clinical science as a foundational field of study has the potential to significantly alter the formation of new physicians. Finding ways to attend to HSS with vigor and inquiry equivalent to that of the clinical and basic sciences surfaces as a challenge. Value-added medical education, properly envisioned and planned, has the capacity to meet that challenge. Such education involves experiential roles for students in practice environments that have the likelihood of positively impacting individual patient and population health outcomes, costs of care, or other processes within the health system while also enhancing student knowledge, attitudes, and skills in the clinical or basic sciences. Kotter's change management framework and Kern's six steps of curriculum development offer lenses to aid in the creation of value-added roles for learners to authentically contribute to patient care while also to discover experientially the tenets of HSS. The first three steps of Kern's and Kotter's frameworks lay the foundation for revolutionizing medical education to include learning opportunities for students in value-added roles.

INTRODUCTION

In his 1910 report entitled "Medical Education in the United States and Canada," Abraham Flexner put forth a framework for medical education consisting of 2 years of basic sciences and 2 years of clinical training based on scientific inquiry and discovery rather than past traditions and practices.[1] Flexner's two-pillar model improved the level of excellence in medical schools over the course of the 20th century, yet the environment in which our clinicians now provide care has markedly changed. With that change, the skills of our clinicians must also evolve.[1] Current challenges in our medical education system include poor understanding of the nonclinical roles of physicians and inadequate attention to the skills required for effective team-delivered care in a complex health care system.[1]

The 2010 book *Educating Physicians: A Call for Reform of Medical School and Residency* presents an update to Flexner's work, making recommendations for enhancing medical education in light of the need for competence in educating, advocating, innovating, investigating, and managing teams.[1] Toward this goal, we assert that for students to prepare for and integrate these roles and skills, their learning in basic, clinical, and health systems sciences should be integrated with their clinical experiences.[1] Learners should have opportunities to experience the broader professional roles of physicians, such as educator, advocate, and investigator; interprofessional teamwork should be incorporated into the medical education curriculum; and learners should participate authentically in inquiry, innovation, and improvement of care.[1]

An emerging three-pillar framework of undergraduate medical education furthers this integration in which HSS is allied with basic science and clinical science as a field of study attended to with equal vigor and inquiry.[2,3] HSS is the study of how health care is delivered, how health care professionals work together to deliver that care, and how the health system can improve patient care and health care delivery.[3] This third pillar of education encompasses health care policy, health systems improvement, population health, interprofessional teamwork, and behavioral and social determinants of health.[2,3] This chapter discusses how students may serve in value-added medical education while also learning about HSS.

As defined earlier in this volume and in the work of Jed Gonzalo and his team at Penn State College of Medicine: "Value-added medical education involves experiential roles for students in practice environments that have the potential to positively impact individual patient and population health outcomes, costs of care, or other processes within the health system, while also enhancing student knowledge, attitudes, and skills in the clinical or HSS."[4] Students are well situated to add value to the health system in that they have time, technology-related skills, and fresh eyes.[5] Students bring a beginner's mind and fresh eyes to the health system; their inquiry may benefit teamwork and patient care through discussion, analysis, and quality improvement.[5]

Primary care clerkships, a staple of clinical learning for medical students, have struggled to retain quality clinical training sites due to time constraints, productivity demands, competition for a limited number of training sites, physicians' concerns about their ability to be effective teachers, physician burnout, and outdated practice models.[6,7] Striving to integrate students into clinical work in useful and authentic ways is one strategy developed to address the concern of retaining quality clinical sites.[6] Tasks such as medication reconciliation, providing patient education, drawing blood, and administering vaccines are all examples of possible value-added roles in clinical care, in which the learner brings value to the clinical setting while authentically contributing to patient care.[8,9] By finding creative and innovative ways for students to add value to outpatient care, preceptors may feel that teaching is more desirable in that this approach may lessen the time investment required to teach while also helping students to learn in a more active and engaged manner.[8]

Another opportunity is to add quality improvement projects to the curriculum.[10] Performing quality improvement projects from start to finish with emergency department physicians provided a unique value-added learning experience; students felt empowered to make positive change and felt they were able to work as colleagues while learning key research skills of data collection, critical analysis, and academic writing.[10] Students want to contribute authentically and be vital members of the team.

In developing medical education curriculum and learning strategies, many medical educators use Kern's six steps of curriculum development.[11] The *Guidebook for Clerkship Directors* by the Alliance for Clinical Education encourages clerkship directors to consider the change management needed to ensure successful and lasting improvement efforts because making change in health care systems requires an understanding of the processes, context, culture, people, and technology within each system.[12] Kotter offers eight steps that can be used for successful change management.[13] These two models intersect to provide a substantial framework to build medical education programming in which medical students perform value-added roles in HSS.[2] We focus this chapter on HSS through the lens of Kern's and Kotter's frameworks toward developing value-added roles in medical education (Fig. 11.1).

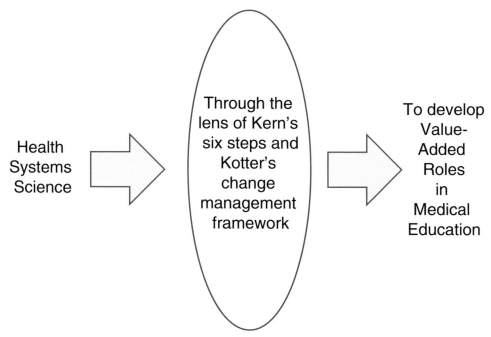

Fig. 11.1 In this chapter, we are looking at HSS through the lens of Kern's six steps and Kotter's change management framework to develop value-added roles in medical education.

KERN'S CURRICULUM DEVELOPMENT APPROACH

Kern's six-step approach to curriculum development posits that medical education curricula should be linked to health care needs.[11] The approach stems from four key beliefs: (1) educational programs should have aims or goals; (2) medical educators are professionally and ethically obligated to meet the needs of learners, patients, and society; (3) medical educators should be held accountable for the outcomes of their interventions; and (4) a logical, systematic approach to curriculum development will contribute to achieving this accountability.[11] The six steps of curriculum development are outlined in Fig. 11.2. They include problem identification and general needs assessment, targeted needs assessment, goals and objectives, educational strategies, implementation, and evaluation and feedback.[11] These steps do not need to occur sequentially or linearly and are more likely to occur in a dynamic, interactive process.[11] Further, curriculum development never really ends. Rather, the curriculum should be refined on an ongoing basis, based on evaluations and changes in resources, learners, and skills.[11]

KOTTER'S CHANGE MANAGEMENT FRAMEWORK

Kotter's change management framework describes the eight steps to produce a successful change of any magnitude in organizations. The eight steps are outlined in Fig. 11.2 and are (1) establish a sense of urgency, (2) create the guiding coalition, (3) develop a vision and strategy, (4) communicate the change vision, (5) empower a broad base of people to take action, (6) generate short-term wins, (7) consolidate gains and produce even more change, and (8) institutionalize new approaches in the culture.[13] The first four steps build a foundation for the sought-after cultural change to occur in an organization. The fifth, sixth, and seventh steps are the action steps in change management in which new practices are introduced, and the eighth step cements the new changes into the culture of the organization.[13] In contrast to the nonsequential nature of Kern's six steps, Kotter notes that change management must occur through eight sequential, linear stages and that "skipping even a single step or getting too far ahead without a solid base almost always creates problems."[13] Kotter also emphasizes that effective change management relies on leadership

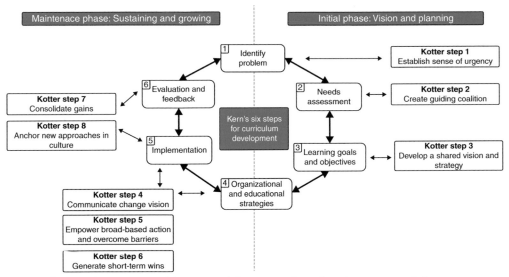

Fig. 11.2 Synthetic conceptual framework for curriculum development and change management when building new partnerships between medical education and health systems. The inner circle reflects Kern's six-step approach to curriculum development; the outer boxes reflect the eight steps in Kotter's change management model. The initial phase reflects the vision and planning phase of medical education–health system partnerships and aligns Kern's steps 1–3 with Kotter's steps 1–3. The maintenance phase reflects the sustaining and growing phase of these new partnerships and aligns Kern's steps 4–5 with Kotter's steps 4–6 and Kern's steps 5–6 with Kotter's steps 7–8. (Reprinted with permission from Gonzalo JD, Lucey C, Wolpaw T, Chang A. Value-added clinical systems learning roles for medical students that transform education and health: a guide for building partnerships between medical schools and health systems. *Acad Med.* 2017;92(5):602–607.)

rather than management skills and defines leadership as a set of processes that creates organizations or adapts organizations to significantly changing circumstances.[13] Hence, this framework can be used to change the culture of medical education in these shifting times to integrate the principles of HSS as tenets of core medical education.

VISION AND PLANNING

Today's physicians must learn the principles of HSS just as they learn about the basic and clinical sciences. Kotter's change management framework and Kern's six steps of curriculum development offer lenses through which HSS may be viewed in order to create value-added roles for learners to authentically contribute to patient care while also experientially discovering the tenets of HSS. We have combined the first three steps of Kern's and Kotter's frameworks to lay the foundation for revolutionizing medical education to include learning opportunities for students in value-added

roles. Our Step 1 combines Kern's first step of identifying the problem with Kotter's recommendation of establishing a sense of urgency. Step 2 melds Kern's step of conducting a needs assessment with Kotter's recommendation of creating the guiding coalition. Step 3 merges Kern's step of identifying learning goals and objectives and Kotter's recommendation of developing a shared vision and strategy. Our rapidly changing health care environment demands that physicians be up to the tasks at hand, ready to competently apply a variety of new skills. Kotter's change management stages are especially applicable and useful for such a metamorphosing delivery system; change management skills are less needed in a stable, consistent setting.[13] Kern's model allows medical educators to quickly respond to a dynamically evolving milieu on an ongoing basis.[11] Together, the combined first three steps of these two models lay the groundwork for a major cultural shift among educators with the vision and planning necessary to integrate HSS into medical education.

Step 1: Establish a Sense of Urgency and Identify the Problem

This first step of problem identification is foundational for curriculum development. All of the other steps depend on having a clear understanding of the problem.[11] Step 1 is also vital in that it supports the generalizability of the curriculum and provides support for that curriculum.[11] Likewise, Step 1 of Kotter's change management model—establish a sense of urgency—is foundational in that without a sense of urgency, transformation is less likely to be successful. Without some compelling reason, stakeholders may not be willing to embrace the sacrifices, cooperation, and initiative required for change to occur.[13] By becoming an expert in the area of the identified need, the medical educator will be better able to create and communicate a sense of urgency for curricular change.[13]

So, let us model this initial step. What is the problem here? Why are we discussing the need for value-added roles in medical education? Rapid changes in health care policy initiatives, payment models, health care delivery systems, and health information technology, data, and informatics are rapidly changing how health care is provided and paid for in the US.[3] With increasing productivity demands, schools are challenged in retaining quality clinical faculty.[2,6] In addition to being able to communicate with patients, critically consider diagnoses and determine best management options; today's physician must also understand the complex process systems on which each patient encounter is based.[3] Policy and systems leaders have expressed that physicians are not being adequately prepared with the necessary HSS skills for optimal functioning in this changing health care environment.[2] Further, physicians must also become health care change agents as collaborators and leaders in changing health care systems with self-transforming minds.[3] Those with self-transforming minds have the abilities to mediate conflicts, review and integrate input from various perspectives, perceive situations in context, and lead flexibly through change and uncertainty.[3]

The need for students to learn about HSS is clear, yet experiential learning opportunities are uncommon.[2] Ideally, students could learn about HSS firsthand through longitudinal, meaningful value-added roles (such as patient navigator, health coach, and panel manager) and tasks (such as performing medication reconciliation, writing drafts of after-visit summaries, calling patients after discharge, and collecting data for quality improvement projects).[2] In addition to learning about HSS, by serving in these value-added roles and through performing these tasks, students would also be necessary members of the health care team.[3] Being a true contributor to the health care team and acquiring a deep understanding of the roles

and tasks of interprofessional health care colleagues fosters not only HSS learning but also professional development.[3]

Just as Kern's first step of problem identification requires a scholarly approach to seek out all necessary information, Kotter suggests that one method for initiating quality efforts is to provide employees with information about problems, potential problems, and potential opportunities.[11,13] This complete review must include accrediting standards and current methods of assessment.[11] Standard 7 of the LCME Standards for Accreditation states that medical school faculty should ensure that the core curriculum of the medical education program prepares medical students to function collaboratively on health care teams that include health professionals from other disciplines as they provide coordinated services to patients.[14] The Physician Competency Reference Set (PCRS), created in 2013 by the Association of American Medical Colleges (AAMC), is a list of common learner expectations utilized in the training of physicians that includes several HSS competencies related to systems-based practice and interprofessional collaboration.[15] The sixth domain of the PCRS emphasizes that students should demonstrate an awareness of and responsiveness to the larger context and system of health care and that students should develop the ability to call effectively on other resources in the system to provide optimal health care. The seventh domain encourages learners to demonstrate the ability to engage in an interprofessional team in a manner that optimizes safe, effective patient- and population-centered care.[15]

Furthermore, the AAMC's entrustable professional activities, or EPAs, are a list of 13 vital tasks that incoming interns should be entrustable with on day one of internship. Several of these involve HSS-related skills: EPA 8, give or receive a patient handover to transition care responsibility; EPA 9, collaborate as a member of an interprofessional team; EPA 11, obtain informed consent for tests and/or procedures; and EPA 13, identify system failures and contribute to a culture of safety and improvement.[16]

Meeting these AAMC standards and EPAs can be daunting. Seeing these accreditation elements alongside the lack of HSS experiential learning opportunities within many of our current evolving health care delivery systems and environments reinforces the urgency of this situation. In this challenge, an opportunity can be found in the possibility of students learning about HSS experientially by serving in integral roles and providing value-added care.

Step 2: Create the Guiding Coalition and Conduct a Needs Assessment

In Step 2 of Kern's model for developing curriculum, medical educators perform a targeted needs assessment to identify the specific needs of their particular learners in their particular learning environment.[11] For instance, where in the current curriculum are students already learning about HSS in the classroom and in the clinical setting? Clerkship directors planning an HSS curriculum should learn which HSS-related curricula students have participated in prior to each clerkship.[12] Faculty may also search school curriculum databases for HSS topics in the curriculum for horizontal and vertical integration.[12]

In this step, stakeholders are involved in the process of solution seeking and addressing the problem identified in Step 1.[11] Relationship building with participating parties helps align resources, clarify problems and opportunities, set goals, and provide insight.[11] In addition to the usually considered stakeholders in medical education—learners, course or clerkship directors, program directors, faculty, and accrediting bodies—when considering HSS learning needs, hospital and interprofessional leaders should also be included. A strong guiding coalition is vital for successful change management; one person cannot sustain the process.[13] This guiding coalition ideally consists of appropriate stakeholders with sufficient trust and shared sense of the problems, objectives, opportunities, and commitment to change.[13] While no individual has all of the data required for decision-making or the time and credibility to convince others to implement decisions, a guiding coalition of stakeholders allows for the collection of all of the information needed to make appropriate, responsive decisions in a situation in flux, while also contributing the time and credibility needed toward the change process.[13] Such a coalition can also speed up the implementation of transformative processes, because strong stakeholders are invested in and committed to key decisions.[13]

By first building relationships with educators and health systems leaders and then initiating key conversations, the foundation for a guiding coalition can begin.[2] These conversations should include health systems leaders from affiliates and community partners such as deans, chief executive officers, chief quality officers, or chief operating officers and include medical educators such as education or curriculum deans.[2] This advisory board should also include members from varied professions, specialties, and sites.[2] Other stakeholders who should be consulted include patients and learners.[5] Medical educators should also work closely with acting internship directors and faculty responsible for transitioning students to residency, as well as core specialty graduate medical education residency program directors to ensure that graduates begin internships with the knowledge, skills, and attitudes required for successful HSS efforts as residents.[12] Such a team of clinical and health systems leaders contributes to the design of education programs within those health systems by identifying specific problems and solution strategies, system needs, and goals for a shared vision.[2]

Step 3: Develop a Shared Vision and Strategy and Identify Learning Goals and Objectives

In Step 3 of Kern's framework for developing curriculum, the focus is on the setting of broad goals and specific measurable learning objectives.[11] Broad educational goals communicate the overall purposes of the curriculum while also serving as criteria for choosing specific learning activities and assessments.[11] Asking for input from stakeholders—such as learners, content experts, interprofessional team members, and health systems leaders—ensures that the specific HSS learning objectives are properly communicated.[11] It is important to find a balance in writing the learning objectives so that they are not so exhaustive as to be overwhelming but are also not so brief as to provide little distinct direction.[11]

Broad goals provide the desired overall direction for a curriculum.[11] Through the development of these overarching goals, educators can develop a shared vision.[13] These common goals should be both sensible to the head and appealing to the heart.[13] A good vision clarifies the direction of change, motivating and aligning people to move in that direction.[13]

Through the development and communication of a shared vision and specific objectives, medical education leaders can effectively partner with health systems leaders toward teaching HSS via value-added roles.[2] Through effective teamwork, the guiding coalition revises the shared vision over time so that it remains desirable, feasible, focused, flexible, and conveyable.[13] While the goal of this chapter is to discuss how curriculum can be planned for students to learn experientially about HSS, curriculum planning may not be part of the shared vision for each individual affiliate or health system. The guiding coalition can tailor a generalized ideal into a more individualized vision that makes more sense for each site and its culture. If the overall vision is for medical trainees to better understand the various ways that health care is delivered, how patients receive care, and how health systems work, how does this idea play out as a shared vision at specific sites?

One example of broad goals in medical education can be found in the Society of Teachers of Family Medicine National Clerkship Curriculum.[17] The curriculum starts off by laying out that the overarching purpose of the family medicine clerkship is to provide foundational knowledge and skill acquisition pertinent to the practice of family medicine to all medical students.[17] The report then lists six learning objectives that students should be able to achieve by the end of their family medicine clerkship. One of these is HSS related: students should be able to discuss the critical role of family physicians within any health care system.[17] Based on the broad goal of understanding the role of family physicians, more specific learning objectives help the student to learn that health systems based on primary care, compared with those not based on primary care, have better medical outcomes, lower medical costs, improved access, and decreased health disparities.[17]

VALUE-ADDED EXAMPLES FROM THE COVID-19 PANDEMIC

The COVID-19 pandemic provides many examples of the responsibilities that medical students can take on in value-added roles while learning directly about HSS.[18] The AAMC recommended that medical students not participate in direct patient contact activities during the early stages of the COVID-19 pandemic for the safety of students and in response to the lack of personal protective equipment.[19,20] Medical educators and students quickly morphed their daily tasks to respond to the demands of this pandemic, with students stepping into HSS roles and tasks and learning about HSS while contributing greatly to the demands that the pandemic placed on the health care system.

For example, students at the University of Colorado School of Medicine worked in call centers, fielding questions about people's symptoms and when to get tested or go to the hospital.[21] At Florida International University Herbert Wertheim College of Medicine, medical students worked in pairs to telephone homeless patients in quarantine in hotel rooms daily to check on their symptoms and refer to a physician or hospital when necessary.[22] At the University of Minnesota, faculty designed curriculum for third and fourth year students during their medical intensive care unit rotation to assist in HSS roles to help the health system to best respond to the COVID-19 pandemic.[23] Students utilized triage protocols to assist with patient placement, review patient charts, and craft detailed summaries for physicians and other health professionals to review and approve, in order to help with transfers and discharges.[23] By writing initial drafts of transfer and discharge summaries, students helped to reduce the amount of time that physicians needed to spend on this necessary task.[23] Medical students also collaborated with pharmacy students on discharge medication, reconciliation, and pharmaceutical literature about treatments for COVID-19.[23]

The Contact Tracing Task Force at Penn State College of Medicine provides another example of experiential learning about HSS while serving in a value-added role.[24] The shared vision of this task force is to mitigate the impact of COVID-19 on the community through the specific strategies of contact tracing, onboarding new contact tracers, and identifying recovered COVID patients willing to donate plasma containing antibodies, which are being studied as a possible treatment for patients hospitalized with COVID-19.[24] Students also identify and share resources for quarantined individuals to help alleviate barriers some patients may face in accessing groceries or medications while quarantined at home.[24] Leading this task force is Dr. Chris Sciamanna, professor of medicine and public health sciences, who notes that the creation of this task force has the potential to support the health care system and provide experiential opportunities for students to learn key concepts such as teamwork, interprofessional collaboration, and social determinants of health.[24]

This rapid evolution in curriculum elegantly demonstrates how medical students can effectively bring value to the health system in times of great need while also learning important foundational skills that will further their training as rounded physicians with solid understandings of the three pillars of medical education. While this chapter has focused on deliberate planning over time in order to retain preceptors while providing vital learning to students, these COVID-19-related examples demonstrate that value-added roles in HSS may be instigated rapidly in response to changing health situations. Through vision and planning, these efforts have been implemented quickly in a way that benefits health systems, medical students, and—most importantly—patients.

CONCLUSION

It is vital that medical students learn about health systems science (HSS) as a foundational field of study with equal robustness as they learn the basic and clinical sciences. By utilizing value-added medical education, in which students gain experiential knowledge in practice environments, students may have positive impacts on individual patient and population health outcomes, on costs of care, and on other processes within the health system. Kotter's change management framework and Kern's six steps of curriculum development offer lenses to aid in the creation of value-added roles for learners to authentically contribute to patient care while also discovering experientially the tenets of HSS. The next chapter continues in this exploration of using Kern's and Kotter's frameworks to transform medical education to include learning opportunities for students in value-added roles.

TAKE-HOME POINTS

- The emerging three-pillar framework of an undergraduate medical education in which health systems science is allied with basic science and clinical science as a foundational field of study has the potential to significantly alter the formation of new physicians.

- Value-added medical education, properly envisioned and planned, has the capacity to meet the challenge of finding ways to attend to health systems science with vigor and inquiry equivalent to that of the basic and clinical sciences.
- Value-added education involves experiential roles for students in practice environments that have the likelihood of positively impacting individual patient and population health outcomes, costs of care, or other processes within the health system while also enhancing student knowledge, attitudes, and skills in the clinical or basic sciences.
- Kotter's change management framework and Kern's six steps of curriculum development offer lenses to aid in the creation of value-added roles for learners to authentically contribute to patient care while also to discover experientially the tenets of health systems science.

QUESTIONS FOR FURTHER THOUGHT

1. What is health systems science, and why is this an important topic for future physicians to learn?
2. How can value-added roles in health systems science enhance patient care?
3. How can Kotter's change management and Kern's curriculum development steps be applied to craft curriculum, including value-added roles in health systems science?

REFERENCES

1. Cooke M, Irby DM, O'Brien BC. *Educating Physicians: A Call for Reform of Medical School and Residency*. San Francisco, CA: Jossey-Bass; 2010.
2. Gonzalo JD, Lucey C, Wolpaw T, Chang A. Value-added clinical systems learning roles for medical students that transform education and health: a guide for building partnerships between medical schools and health systems. *Acad Med*. 2017;92(5):602–607.
3. Skochelak SE, Hawkins RE, Lawson LE, Starr SR, Borkan JM, Gonzalo JD. *Health Systems Science*. Philadelphia, PA: Elsevier; 2017.
4. Gonzalo JD, Thompson BM, Haidet P, Mann K, Wolpaw DR. A constructive reframing of student roles and systems learning in medical education using a communities of practice lens. *Acad Med*. 2017;92(12):1687–1694.
5. Gonzalo JD, Dekhtyar M, Hawkins RE, Wolpaw DR. How can medical students add value? Identifying roles, barriers, and strategies to advance the value of undergraduate medical education to patient care and the health system. *Acad Med*. 2017;92(9):1294–1301.
6. Society of Teachers of Family Medicine. Report on the Summit to Address the Shortage of High Quality Primary Care Community Preceptors. https://www.stfm.org/

media/1358/precepting-summit-executive-summary.pdf. Published 2016. Accessed January 12, 2021.
7. Minor S, Huffman M, Lewis P, Kost A, Prunuske J. The CoPPRR Study: community preceptor perspectives about recruitment and retention. *Fam Med*. 2019;51(5):389–398. https://journals.stfm.org/familymedicine/2019/may/minor-2018-0358/. Accessed January 12, 2021.
8. Society of Teachers of Family Medicine Medical Student Education Committee. Strategies to Ensure That Students Add Value in Outpatient Clinics. https://stfm.org/media/1348/studentsasaddedvalue2018.pdf. Published 2018. Accessed January 12, 2021.
9. Graziano SC, McKenzie ML, Abbott JF, et al. Barriers and Strategies to Engaging Our Community-Based Preceptors. *Teach Learn Med*. 2018;30(4):444–450.
10. Pandian HS, Iyer PS, Bhangra JK, Nijhawan A. Introducing medical student-led quality improvement projects as a value-added learning opportunity in the emergency department. *AEM Educ Train*. 2019;3(3):301–302.
11. Kern DE, Thomas PA, Hughes MT. *Curriculum Development for Medical Education: A Six-Step Approach*. 3rd ed. Baltimore, MD: Johns Hopkins University Press; 2016.
12. Morgenstern BZ. *Alliance for Clinical Education Guidebook for Clerkship Directors*. 5th ed. North Syracuse, NY: Gegensatz Press; 2019.
13. Kotter JP. *Leading Change*. Boston, MA: Harvard Business Review Press; 2012.
14. Liaison Committee on Medical Education. Functions and Structure of a Medical School: Standards for Accreditation of Medical Education Programs Leading to the M.D. Degree. https://lcme.org/wp-content/uploads/filebase/standards/2020-21 Functions-and-Structure_2020 11-2. docx. Published March 2020. Accessed June 20, 2020.
15. Association of American Medical Colleges. CI Physician Competency Reference Set (PCRS). https://www.aamc.org/what-we-do/mission-areas/medical-education/curriculum-inventory/establish-your-ci/physician-competency-reference-set. Published 2013. Accessed January 12, 2021.
16. Association of American Medical Colleges. Core Entrustable Professional Activities for Entering Residency: Curriculum Developer's Guide. https://store.aamc.org/downloadable/download/sample/sample_id/63/%20. Published 2014. Accessed January 12, 2021.
17. Society of Teachers of Family Medicine. National Clerkship Curriculum, 2nd edition. https://www.stfm.org/media/1828/ncc_2018edition.pdf. Published 2018. Accessed January 12, 2021.
18. Long N, Wolpaw DR, Boothe D, et al. Contributions of health professions students to health system needs during the COVID-19 pandemic. *Acad Med*. 2020;95(11):1679–1686. https://doi.org/10.1097/acm.0000000000003611.
19. Association of American Medical Colleges. Important Guidance for Medical Students on Clinical Rotations During the Coronavirus (COVID-19) Outbreak. https://www.aamc.org/news-insights/press-releases/important-guidance-medical-students-clinical-rotations-during-coronavirus-covid-19-outbreak. Published March 17, 2020. Accessed January 12, 2021.

20. Association of American Medical Colleges. Guidance on Medical Students' Participation in Direct In-Patient Contact Activities. https://www.aamc.org/system/files/2020-04/meded-April-14-Guidance-on-Medical-Students-Participation-in-Direct-Patient-Contact-Activities.pdf. Published April 14, 2020. Accessed January 12, 2021.

21. Krieger P, Goodnough A. Medical Students, Sidelined for Now, Find New Ways to Fight Coronavirus. *New York Times*. March 23, 2020. https://www.nytimes.com/2020/03/23/health/medical-students-coronavirus.html Accessed January 12, 2021.

22. Varela I. Medical Students Are Helping the Homeless in Quarantine Survive the Virus, Isolation. *FIU News*. June 16, 2020. https://news.fiu.edu/2020/how-fiu-medical-students-are-helping-the-homeless-in-quarantine-survive-the-virus-and-isolation. Accessed January 12, 2021.

23. Atkins K. New Curriculum Equips U of M Medical Students to Support COVID-19 Efforts. *University of Minnesota News and Events*. April 3, 2020. https://med.umn.edu/news-events/new-curriculum-equips-u-m-medical-students-support-covid-19-efforts. Accessed January 12, 2021.

24. Koetter P, Pelton M, Gonzalo J, et al. Implementation and process of a COVID-19 contact tracing initiative: leveraging health professional students to extend the workforce during a pandemic. *Am J Infect Control*. 2020;48(12):1451–1456. https://doi.org/10.1016/j.ajic.2020.08.012.

12

Launching and Sustaining Value-Added Roles

*Carol A. Terregino, Deborah Ziring,
Rosalyn Maben-Feaster, and Maya Hammoud*

LEARNING OBJECTIVES

1. Identify practical approaches to developing value-added systems learning roles that meet curricular objectives and further health system priorities.
2. Discuss the importance of using change-management strategies to generate buy-in and inspire action.
3. List concrete strategies for overcoming obstacles during implementation and for empowering learners in their value-added roles.

OUTLINE

CHAPTER SUMMARY

This chapter explores the operational implementation of programs to create value-added clinical roles. We outline the elements of programs that meet both educational and health system objectives, change-management strategies to generate buy-in and inspire action from stakeholders, and some practical strategies to navigate obstacles and empower our learners. We frame practical considerations in the context of characteristics of successful partnerships, lessons learned from newer partnerships, and strategies to overcome resistance to change in both medical education institutions and health systems.

INTRODUCTION

To be accountable as medical educators and health systems leaders, we must provide learning opportunities "to mobilise knowledge and to engage in critical reasoning and ethical conduct so that they are competent to participate in patient and population-centred health systems as members of locally responsive and globally connected teams."[1]

Achieving this type of accountability to population health outcomes for our learners and the institutions that educate them necessitates a transformation from the traditional roles of medical students as observers practicing skills, participating in service-learning, or functioning as "doctors" in student-run clinics to those who add value to health systems and the populations they serve.[2] Similarly, the roles of medical educators and health system leaders must evolve to those of partners and collaborators whose future success is inextricably intertwined. **Value-added clinical systems learning** roles take us a step further and necessitate a reworking of the medical educator/health system roles, beginning with development of open lines of communication, shared priorities and goal setting, and navigation through challenges.

THEORETICAL FRAMEWORK

Theory

Gonzalo et al.[3] operationalize a model to prepare medical students to be "systems-ready" and active in improving the health of their patients, framed by Kern's curriculum development approach[4] and Kotter's leading organizational change approach.[5] Fusing of these seemingly disparate approaches provides a framework for managing disruption to the status quo in order to successfully achieve the objectives sought. Kotter's Steps 4 and 5—communication of change vision and overcoming barriers and empowering action—and Kern's Step 4—organizational and educational strategies—necessitate a thoughtful presentation of the vision that engages stakeholders in both medical education and clinical roles. That vision should involve the C-suite of the health system and encourage both clinicians and medical educators to identify common objectives while co-constructing a plan of action that anticipates challenges and contains a mechanism for continuous quality improvement. This approach requires top-down, bottom-up, and cross-entity leadership. The importance of mutual respect and the establishment of common goals is no less important than the development of a therapeutic alliance, co-constructing a medical history, or shared decision-making in patient care. Communication of this change vision requires a clear articulation of the meaning of "value-added, determined by what means, by what metric, for whom."

Review of Literature of Health System/Education/ Community Partnerships and Systems-Thinking for Value-Added Roles

Graduate medical education began to tackle the concept of value-added roles earlier, propelled by the clinical learning environment review of the Accreditation Council for Graduate Medical Education (ACGME),[6] which provides a lens to evaluate the intersection of education and the health system where learning occurs. In practice, even though resident learners are paid members of the workforce, the prevailing model has been two parallel entities, the health system and medical education, independently pursuing quality improvement and patient safety. Gupta and Arora[7] describe four processes through which synergies between education and the health system can be realized: alignment of priorities, data-driven decision making, engagement of hospital staff and learners in joint projects, and accountability and incentivization for alignment.

For undergraduate medical education, the literature supports multiple "learning" benefits for medical students in service learning community partnership experiences. A systematic review of service learning in medical education highlighted the educational benefits in terms of skills gained: leadership, communication, self-confidence, and efficacy as well as an understanding the social determinants of health. However, it also acknowledged that rigorous study of community outcomes is needed in order to ensure the "reciprocity" in service learning.[8] A recent student perspective highlights the need to develop holistic approaches to evaluating student contributions to health system improvements.[9]

Review of Literature on Overcoming Resistance in Medical Education and Health Systems

In a compelling 2019 commentary, Wartman provides practical guidelines to address resistance to change in curricular reform. Institutions must ask themselves: Are we "currently educating students to be maximally effective 21st-century practitioners"?[10] He calls upon taking "advantage of the strategic synergies that can arise by creating a virtuous cycle connecting education with research and patient care in a continuous feedback loop" and notes that "in many institutions, these connections are not sufficiently prioritized, with the result that medical schools fail to take advantage of a powerful dynamic whereupon each component regularly improves the performance of the others." Similarly, the health system fails to take advantage of the academic partnership to advance common goals and prepare the 21st-century workforce. There are countless anecdotes of failed educational initiatives due to the failure to collaborate with our health system counterparts. For partnerships to successfully reimagine and implement change, each entity must galvanize change management processes. Pragmatic approaches identified for medical educators[11] are applicable to education–health system partnerships, including identification and prioritization of stakeholder interest and close monitoring of the organizational climate and readiness for change.

A group of medical education experts identified potential barriers to implementation of value-based roles for medical students from student to faculty to health system. They proposed strategies to overcome barriers to current health system design, including alignment of education and health system mission and values, collaboration with the health system on care models that support teams, continuity and relationship building, and broad dissemination of the new education and health system goals to all stakeholders.[2] Even when we can all articulate benefits to learners and work toward achieving the Triple Aim, if we do not build relationships and keep lines of communication open between educators, health system providers and leaders, and our learners, best intentions will fail.

Program Development: Partnerships

Several medical schools have successfully partnered with health systems and communities in the development of value-added roles. Highly successful partnerships occur when there is a detailed plan with clear steps communicating the vision, an outline for overcoming barriers and empowering action, and the means for developing organizational and educational strategies.

Communication of Change Vision

In *Leading Change*, Kotter argues that the key elements to efficient communication of a vision include simplicity, an illustrative message, discussion in multiple forums, repetition, role modeling from leadership, explanations of inconsistencies, and bidirectional communication.[5] Adherence to these principles ensures that everyone involved (learners, medical educators, health care workers, and health system leadership) can describe the vision and apply it to the activities needed to support its success.

Example

At the University of Michigan Medical School (UMMS), university leaders challenged a multidisciplinary taskforce of experts in health systems science (HSS) content domains to design the framework for integrating HSS into the existing medical education curriculum. The Office of Medical Education appointed an HSS thread leader in 2017 to help execute the charge. The guiding vision is that all UMMS graduates will be able to practice medicine integrating basic and clinical sciences along with HSS to lead positive change for patients and the population as a whole. This vision will be achieved via a cohesive HSS curriculum seamlessly integrated into the existing curriculum over all 4 years. Execution of this vision has required extensive communication as medical education has traditionally been siloed and

HSS content domains have not been emphasized. The HSS thread leader, by necessity, meets regularly with the other longitudinal thread leaders, preclinical curricular leaders, clerkship directors, and directors of the professional development years to explain this vision, obtain feedback, and build collaborative relationships. In addition, to facilitate execution of educational initiatives within these content areas, regular bidirectional communication has occurred with health system leaders in the patient safety and quality departments. The HSS thread leader has also met with various student groups that overlap with the HSS content domains and student council representatives to ensure that all stakeholders understand the vision and solicit feedback. All of these meetings have helped to build a coalition behind the vision.

By creating a clarity and consistency to the vision and building of these relationships, the UMMS has been able to ensure that educational endeavors undertaken are aligned with health system goals and initiatives. One value-added clinical learning role that has come out of this process is the Health Systems Science A3 Project, which is completed by all third-year medical students. Students are divided into teams near the beginning of their third year and partnered with a coach from the Quality Department at Michigan Medicine. Through this team project, students learn more about applying foundational quality improvement knowledge in a practical way through the study of health care system problems or gaps that they have identified during their training at Michigan Medicine. In each group, the students learn how to scope a problem appropriately, describe the current situation, perform a root cause analysis of the problem, and develop a plan of action. Work to develop educational roles that further health care system goals and objectives is ongoing but promising as the stakeholders are engaged and committed to success.

Overcoming Barriers and Empowering Action

Creating consistency around a vision is not enough to facilitate success. Kotter argues that you must also empower those involved to make changes to fit the vision.[4] This involves addressing barriers to success, which can come in the form of structures, skills, systems, and leadership.

Leaders must facilitate skill acquisition for the students and for those who will interact with them in their new roles. In addition, they must anticipate structural or system-related barriers and make plans to address them, including creating a business case for educational and health system leadership if new funding is required to achieve the vision. By being thoughtful about the skills, structure, systems, and leadership required to create these new roles for students, they will be able to empower those involved to execute the vision more efficiently.

Example

McDermott et al.[12] illustrate how the learner is empowered to fulfill value-added roles when the experience is designed to provide structure and facilitate support. They describe Penn State College of Medicine's 9-month HSS curriculum, which began in 2014 and includes a patient navigator role as a component of the course. During this course, students are embedded within existing clinical sites within the institution and are assigned a faculty mentor at the site. The authors describe three cases in which students were able to successfully execute value-added roles. In each case, the students were able to work with faculty at the sites to identify and mitigate issues related to social determinants of health in order to have positive impacts on patients. The paper highlights the importance of adequate leadership and support built into the experiences as success appeared to be directly tied to the relationship between the faculty mentor and the student(s).

IDENTIFYING OPPORTUNITIES FOR VALUE-ADDED ROLES AND NEW PARTNERSHIPS

As educational leaders consider ideas for change and innovation to implement value-added roles at their institutions, they should generate an inventory of options that incorporate ideas from other institutions with successful programs, adaptations of programs done elsewhere, or entirely new ideas. As new ideas are imagined, they are inevitably constrained by the parts, skills, and limits of the time. For example, the iPhone would have been difficult to imagine and would not have succeeded unless the internet was in place. Once the internet was available, incremental improvements and innovations occurred to mobile phone technology to eventually enable the current functionality of our "smart" phones, including GPS, internet searching, and other functions. Scientist Stuart Kauffman coined this theory, the adjacent possible.[13] It is a kind of shadow future near the edges of the present state of things. It helps us to imagine how the present can reinvent itself with the tools and skills currently available. As incremental progress is made, insights occur that feed the discovery process, generating new insights and possibilities. This, in turn, opens up new possibilities utilizing different combinations. According to Steven Johnson, in his book *Where Good Ideas Come From*,[14] the secret to innovation is combining these odds and ends to create something new, amplifying this concept of the adjacent possible.

In considering how to add a program for value-added roles, the adjacent possible concept is useful to help assess what is possible given the opportunities and limits in a school's given context. Although other institutions may have successfully implemented a program, the likelihood of successful implementation at a given site will depend on local factors, including the attitudes, skills, culture, and financial resources specific to the environment. Implementing a program that is in the school's adjacent possible, with the intent to iterate over time while enabling it to build and grow, helps ground plans in what can be successfully achieved initially.

MAKING CRITICAL DECISIONS WHEN DEVELOPING ORGANIZATIONAL AND EDUCATIONAL STRATEGIES

While considering the design and implementation of value-added roles for medical students, educators must thoughtfully consider several initial critical questions. These decisions, with contemplation of the pros and cons for each, are imperative for the successful launch of any such program.

First, will the program be a curricular or noncurricular activity? If it will be curricular, approval and implementation will require adherence to approval processes for curricular activities at your institution as well as alignment with the Liason Committee on Medical Education accreditation standards. Course goals, hours, credits, student assessment plans, remediation if necessary, and mapping to competencies must be thought out similarly to any new curricular endeavor. If it is noncurricular, students will need monitoring, but the program would not count toward curricular time and have much less restrictive governance and assessment requirements. However, lack of dedicated curricular time has been found to be a limiting factor in student attitude and engagement.[15] In addition, the program would require adequate free time for students to engage fully.

Next, will the program be for all students or some? If some, is it some students within the same cohort or is it, for example, only Year 1 students? Preparation for the value-added role that students will be performing along with developmental readiness is imperative to success. If the learning goals of the program are essential for all students and not optional, Gonzalo et al. make the case effectively[16] that it must be for all students while Borkan et al.[17] argue that a more limited approach has the benefit of encountering fewer obstacles and challenges to implement. While both are true, consideration of local context and priorities is necessary to determine the best approach to get started. There are strong arguments that having common student roles and experiences with meaningful contributions to patient care early on are pivotal to the development of professional identity formation.[18] Indeed, a qualitative study at one school regarding HSS content found that student engagement was limited as this work was not aligned with a traditional professional identity for physicians.[19,20]

Third, if curricular, should it be a stand-alone course or part of an integrated course? As a stand-alone course, design and delivery of course content, assessment methods, and course requirements are more easily controlled. If it is part of an integrated course, careful design of the assessment paradigm is critical or students may be able to off-set poor performance in their value-added role with high performance on knowledge exams. This approach could result in lack of competence in the areas linked to the value-added role as well as limit student engagement, with priority given to high-stakes knowledge exams. Integration, though, enables students to make connections with other curricular components and supports the importance of the value-added role.

Whether students will have access to the electronic health record (EHR) during the value-added role is another critical decision. Gonzalo et al. suggest additional practical considerations: proximity of the learning site to the medical school; safety of the neighborhood; presence of interprofessional care teams; availability of a site mentor; authenticity of the roles; target populations; and availability of data and infrastructure.[3] Considerations of infrastructure should include both physical space in the learning areas and technology, such as access to the EHR. Over 80% of students in a cross-sectional survey of 2670 medical students at 9 medical schools indicated that working as part of a team increased their desire to participate in these value-added

roles.[15] Since most communication between health care professionals occurs via the EHR, the students' ability to view and document in the EHR enables them to communicate with the team, validating their contributions to patient care. The logistics and permissions within the health care system where students are performing these value-added roles may be a significant barrier to this option and must be discussed with health system leadership to ensure that they are in accordance with policies and meet regulatory requirements around documentation.

Once educational leadership makes these decisions and determines the details of implementation, a list of resources with an accompanying inventory of items that will come from repurposing staff, space, or other items with elements that are already in place will be most beneficial. This list should include a summary of any problems that have been identified and the analysis that has been conducted. It should provide a review of the potential options, a rationale for the option chosen, details of the operational plan, and an outline of the projected financial need.

EXECUTION AT YOUR HOME INSTITUTION

Lessons Learned

Medical schools in the American Medical Association (AMA) Accelerating Change in Medical Education Consortium are at various stages of implementation of value-added roles for medical students. We share three vignettes highlighting the impact of people, operations, and strategy on the ultimate success of programs.

BOX 12.1   Consortium School: Sidney Kimmel Medical College at Thomas Jefferson University

The Importance of People: "Third Time's the Charm."
In 2017, the school launched a value-added roles program for 275 first-year medical students at 7 Jefferson clinical sites. The vision for the program was to provide an experiential component for the health systems science thread content delivered in the didactic curriculum. The goals were for students to work with patients to address underlying social and environmental factors that impact health. This experience would give students the opportunity to actively participate in care and to reflect on the systems and approaches helpful in optimizing health. A director for this course was hired along with an educational coordinator, a social worker, and four community health workers. The inaugural director had earned an MPH and had extensive community outreach and population health research experience at Jefferson, while all other hires were new. The team struggled to form a cohesive unit, complicated by systems issues of being an academic affairs team functioning in seven different clinical environments. Academic leadership also underestimated the need for the director to understand the clinical workflows for successful implementation at some of the sites. This conflict resulted in

Continued

BOX 12.1 Consortium School: Sidney Kimmel Medical College at Thomas Jefferson University—cont'd

marginalization of the students and two sites withdrawing from participation over the initial few months of the program. In addition, as the director of this course was not a physician, there was some lack of student buy-in. They perceived this work as belonging to social workers or public health leaders but not physicians. Despite multiple attempts to problem-solve, it became clear that a change in director leadership was urgently required to salvage this program. It was painful and many felt we should abandon this effort altogether, but our academic leaders were committed to the importance of this curricular experience. The replacement director was a well-respected primary care physician, with an MD and MPH, who "walked the walk." During this second year, major wins included having sites participate in workflow development and having students granted access to the EHR, where they documented patient encounters. Buy-in from students and sites improved, but this director resigned after that year to relocate. As the school considered new candidates, they realized that success in this role was less about content knowledge and more about communication skills, problem-solving ability, and systems-level thinking. For the third director, the school hired an emergency medicine physician with design-thinking experience, strong interpersonal and communication skills, and systems-level relationships. He has been wildly successful in this role, creating alliances across the enterprise. Most recently, he has optimized the community health workers' remote work as they communicate with COVID-19 patients at these sites. As the program enters its fourth year, the initial vision for this value-added student role has become a reality, with an expanding "adjacent possible," and value-added roles can move forward with the right people in place.

BOX 12.2 Consortium School: Rutgers Robert Wood Johnson Medical School

The Importance of Operations: "Don't Bite Off More Than You Can Chew."

The operational challenges of embedding interprofessional learners on care coordination teams within the structure of an academic clinical partnership and an accountable care organization are daunting. The challenges emphasize the critical role of operations in the implementation phase of any value-added program. Medical/nursing/pharmacy/social work student teams were paired with a nurse care coordinator following a community-dwelling patient with multiple chronic conditions. After the first nurse care coordinator and interprofessional learner team visit, the student teams would independently make home visits with the goal of "adding value" to care coordination. Education leadership underestimated the complexity of operations between school and health system, school and other professional schools, and clinical operations of the school versus the clinical operations of a health system partner. Continuing the theme of the first lessons-learned example that people matter in operations, the education leaders found that some of the care coordinators were not interested in embracing a teaching role and saw the student learners as burdensome. The AMA Accelerating Change in Medical Education Consortium grant team did not fully appreciate the nuances of finances, employees who were spread too thin, and a locus of control at the accountable care organization that would impede the implementation of the educational activities of the consortium grant. The medical school collaborated with leadership at other health professions schools on the home visit project. Nevertheless, numerous logistical issues complicated matters. Lingering questions remained: "Is this for some students or all students?"; "Is this a freestanding experience or one integrated into standard course activities?"; and "What time works for all students, the nurse care coordinator, and, most importantly, the patient?" Even the selection and implementation of a HIPAA-compliant platform that could be used by students, faculty, and employees of the health system proved challenging. The operational demands of learners in value-added roles require a significant investment in infrastructure. The program has posted real wins for most students, some care coordinators, and health system finances. Adding value, however, and achieving large-scale sustainability and dissemination throughout the health professional schools and the accountable care organization was hampered by the operational challenges. Rutgers has currently achieved success with the interprofessional home visit program as a selective for approximately a third of the class, with medical student–pharmacy student teams under the supervision of a family medicine physician in the faculty practice of the medical school.

BOX 12.3   Consortium School: Rutgers Robert Wood Johnson Medical School

The Importance of Strategy: "You Can Never Overcommunicate."

Rutgers Robert Wood Johnson Medical School embarked on another value-added project with the ultimate goal of systematically improving teamwork in the health system by training all medical students and a cadre of faculty and health system staff in TeamSTEPPS (Team Strategies To Enhance Performance and Patient Safety).[21] The school optimistically envisioned medical students in the value-added role of change agents to systematize evidence-based team strategies such as briefing, debriefing, leadership, and communication strategies.[21] Acknowledging the need to prepare students for the health system and future practice, the school made the decision to influence changes in the larger health system rather than relegate this teamwork project to the medical student training environment. The school sought strategies to transform the health system and when devising strategy, underestimated the inertia of the status quo and the resistance it generated. There was a failure to communicate the change vision and implement a project *after* planning with partners and an underestimation of the complexities of the multiple nonlinear, unpredictable, self-organizing forces of a health system. The school failed to fully catalyze the needed cultural change for effective teamwork training.

It was more than just "culture." In order to effectively transform a system and create value-added roles, the medical education program needed to change both institutional culture and *habitus*, a deeply entrenched and difficult-to-change system of embodied dispositions or tendencies that organizes the ways individuals perceive the social world around them and react to it.[22,23] The school aimed to create and sustain a vibrant and respectful learning community of practice but failed to initially co-create a shared vision with the right people. Failure to communicate early and effectively and in both the education and health system arena—including the quality and safety officer—led to a major misunderstanding between concepts of the high-reliability organization and standardized teamwork training (i.e., TeamSTEPPS). The educational leaders and the school faculty were not fully informed that the hospital was embarking on another quality and safety initiative. Faculty were skeptical that any teamwork training could enhance productivity and patient safety. They believed that this training and practice would add one more thing to already full clinical, administrative, and academic loads. There was a lack of staff engagement in using the teamwork strategies following the TeamSTEPPS Master Training course. In retrospect, there were two crucial failures: a failure of educators to co-create the vision with quality and safety leaders at the school and health system and a failure to communicate widely in order to anticipate what could go wrong. These shortfalls resulted in rolling out a value-added project during preparation for Joint Commission accreditation for the outpatient practice, which resulted in competing organizational priorities. The lessons learned informed a new TeamSTEPPS project in the critical care unit with full engagement of undergraduate medical education, graduate medical education, and the health system. The operationalization of this project, which included the value-added roles of students as critical care team members, provided a structured team environment in the intensive care units. The model has subsequently become critical in the management of the COVID-19 surge.

TAKE-HOME POINTS

1. When developing strategic visions for value-added systems learning roles, it is critical to be thoughtful about the opportunities that currently exist and how to align educational objectives for medical students with health system priorities.
2. Once identified, the vision should be concisely and coherently articulated to others. All stakeholder groups should be engaged in adapting the vision and should be able to participate in regular bidirectional communication.
3. It is critical to develop a plan to create the structure, skills, systems, and leadership to support the vision and work with the stakeholders to identify additional barriers and possible solutions in order to help with execution.

4. Operational needs, with adequate infrastructure and human resources, must not be underestimated, and a stable source of funding will offer a greater chance of success for the program.

QUESTIONS FOR FURTHER THOUGHT

1. What techniques will you use to communicate your vision to stakeholders?
2. What resources will you need to obtain or cultivate to achieve success?
3. What obstacles will you need to address to facilitate empowerment toward action?

ANNOTATED BIBLIOGRAPHY

Gonzalo JD, Lucey C, Wolpaw T, Chang A. Value-added clinical systems learning roles for medical students that transform education and health: a guide for building parnerships between medical schools and health systems. *Acad Med*. 2017;92(5):602–607. https://doi.org/10.1097/ACM.000000000001346.

Gonzalo et al. contextualize the creation of new clinical systems learning roles for medical students within the frameworks of Kotter's eight steps for change management and Kern's six steps for curriculum development. The two medical schools, Penn State College of Medicine and University of California, San Francisco, School of Medicine used these frameworks in similar fashion, providing internal validity for developing partnerships between education and clinical enterprises. The eight strategies—from developing a shared mental model between the health system and the education enterprise to implementation, evaluation, and sustainability of these roles and the practical considerations—provide a roadmap for schools considering development of these roles.

Gupta R, Arora VM. Merging the health system and education silos to better educate future physicians. *JAMA*. 2015;314:2349–2350.

In this viewpoint, Gupta and Arora articulate the importance of the clinical learning environment in imprinting behaviors on trainees and outline steps to create synergies between the health system and medical education so that "AMCs can use to accomplish their dual missions of delivering high-quality care and preparing the next generation of physicians for new models of value-based care and population health." They describe "bridging roles" for medical students or residents and discuss the value added by these roles.

REFERENCES

1. Frenk J, Chen L, Bhutta ZA, et al. Health professionals for a new century: transforming education to strengthen health systems in an interdependent world. *Lancet*. 2010;376:1923–1958.
2. Gonzalo JD, Dekhtyar M, Hawkins RE, Wolpaw DR. How can medical students add value? Identifying roles, barriers, and strategies to advance the value of undergraduate medical education to patient care and the health system. *Acad Med*. 2017;92:1294–1301.
3. Gonzalo JD, Lucey C, Wolpaw T, Chang A. Value-added clinical systems learning roles for medical students that transform education and health: a guide for building parnerships between medical schools and health systems. *Acad Med*. 2017;92(5):602–607. https://doi.org/10.1097/ACM.000000000001346.
4. Kern DE, Thomas PA, Hughes MT. *Curriculum Development for Medical Education: A Six-Step Approach*. 2nd ed. Baltimore, MD: Johns Hopkins University Press; 2009.
5. Kotter JP. *Leading Change*. Boston, MA: Harvard Business Review Press; 2012.
6. Accreditation Council for Graduate Medical Education. Clinical Learning Environment (CLER). https://www. acgme.org/What-We-Do/Initiatives/Clinical-Learning-Environment-Review-CLER. Accessed January 13, 2021.
7. Gupta R, Arora VM. Merging the health system and education silos to better educate future physicians. *JAMA*. 2015;314:2349–2350.
8. Stewart T, Wubenna ZC. A systematic review of service-learning in medical education: 1998–2012. *Teach Learn Med*. 2015;27(2):115–122. https://doi.org/10.1080/10401334.2015.1011647.
9. Gylys R, Rosenwohl-Mack S, Pierluissii E, Hoffman A. Assessing contributions of value-added medical student roles. *Med Teach*. 2020. https://doi.org/10.1080/0142159X.2020.1755634.
10. Wartman SA. The empirical challenge of 21st century medical education. *Acad Med*. 2019;94:1412–1415.
11. Edwards RA, Venugopal S, Navedo D, Ramanii S. Addressing needs of diverse stakeholders: twelve tips for leaders of health professionsl education programs. *Med Teach*. 2019;41:17–23.
12. McDermott C, Shank K, Shervinskie C, Gonzalo JD. Developing a professional identity as a change agent early in medical school: the students' voice. *J Gen Intern Med*. 2019;34:750–753.
13. Kauffman S. *At Home in the Universe: The Search for the Laws of Self-Organization and Complexity*. New York, NY: Oxford University Press; 1995.
14. Johnson S. *Where Good Ideas Come From*. New York, NY: Riverhead Books; 2010.
15. Leep Hunderfund AN, Starr SR, Dyrbye LN, Gonzalo JD, Miller GP, Morgan HK, et al. Value-added activities in medical education: a multi-site survey of first- and second-year medical students' perceptions and factors influencing their potential engagement. *Acad Med*. 2018;93:1560–1568.
16. Gonzalo JD, Wolpaw T, Wolpaw D. Curricular transformation in health systems science: the need for global change. *Acad Med*. 2018;93:1431–1433.
17. Borkan JM, George P, Tunkel AR. Curricular transformation: the case against global change. *Acad Med*. 2018;93:1428–1430.
18. Gonzalo JD, Thompson BM, Haidet P, Mann K, Wolpaw DR. A constructive reframing of student roles and systems learning in medical education using a communities of practice lens. *Acad Med*. 2017;92:1687–1694.
19. Gonzalo JD, Davis C, Thompson BM, Haidet P. Unpacking medical students' mixed engagement in health systems science education. *Teach Learn Med*. 2020;32:250–258.
20. Gonzalo JD, Ogrinc G. Health Systems Science: The "broccoli" of undergraduate medical student education. *Acad Med*. 2019;94:1425–1432.
21. Agency for HTeamSTEPPS. https://www.ahrq.gov/teamstepps/index.html. Accessed January 13, 2021.
22. Wikipedia. Habitus. https://en.wikipedia.org/wiki/Habitus. Accessed January 13, 2021.
23. Balmer DF, Richards BF, Varpio L. How students experience and navigate transitions in undergraduate medical education: an application of Bourdieu's theoretical model. *Adv Health Sci Educ Theory Pract*. 2015;20(4):1073–1085.

13

Improving and Growing Value-Added Roles

Jesse M. Ehrenfeld and Brian J. Miller

LEARNING OBJECTIVES

1. Explain an approach to iterating and growing value-added roles over time.
2. Describe barriers to scalable uptake of value-added roles.

3. Identify the importance of anchoring approaches in the culture.

OUTLINE

CHAPTER SUMMARY

In this chapter, we describe long-term sustainability challenges facing medical education, the importance of stakeholder perspectives when integrating value-added roles for students, and strategies to overcome obstacles to long-term adoption and growth of these activities. By understanding the current context and challenges, this chapter and its discussion of change management strategies guides readers toward approaches to growing and sustaining value-added roles.

INTRODUCTION

As policy experts question the federal government's funding of graduate medical education (GME),[1] the downward economic pressure on academic medical centers (AMCs) and health care organizations persists,[2] forcing AMCs and parent health systems to consider new financing and delivery models. With increasing pressure, the traditional protected model of undergraduate medical education (UME) is under attack. AMCs are exploring value-added roles for medical students, expanding the traditional role of UME in order to support dual institutional educational and operational missions. These growing contributions are evolving into an essential component of the value equation that will enable medical education to survive and subsequently thrive, providing medical students new venues for practical learning and growth.

With this framework in mind, in this final chapter we take stock of strategies for improving and growing value-added roles. In keeping with the paradigm offered by Kotter's steps for change management[3] and Kern's steps for curriculum development,[4] we focus on how organizations can generate short-term wins during implementation, consolidate those gains while beginning evaluation and feedback, and ultimately anchor these new educational approaches within an organization's culture.

THE ACADEMIC MEDICAL CENTER: A MODEL UNDER DURESS

The unique mission of the AMC—with its focus on education, patient care, and research—also makes AMCs vulnerable to a variety of external risks. Leaders face a multi-pronged "trial by fire" of financing and operational challenges, external demands for constant improvements in research productivity in the context of investigator difficulties in accessing federal research funding,[5] and changing educational paradigms as medical students and postgraduate trainees increasingly evolve from learners into additional complementary roles as employees[6] and consumers.

AMCs traditionally have some of the highest cost structures for the delivery of complex, specialized care to patients. As there is increasing downward pressure on clinical reimbursement, the embedded costs of running an AMC can put additional strain on the other nonclinical missions: education and research.[7] This is often particularly acute in systems where the payer mix is more heavily weighted toward patients with government-sponsored health insurance (i.e., Medicare and Medicaid), which reimburses at lower rates.[8] These revenue challenges are often further compounded by the inherent issues brought on by the mechanisms by which medical education is financed, at both the UME and GME level. UME financing challenges include the problem of a decades-old system,[9] which relies on a "pay as you go" approach, whereas GME financing challenges center around the fixed federal payments that have not been appropriately recalibrated in many years.[10]

In addition to the financial challenges to creating value-added roles, there are a number of operational considerations unique to AMCs. These include throughput pressure to generate case volumes and increase relative value units (RVUs) given that few centers have meaningfully transitioned to the provision of value-based care by participation in capitated commercial insurance models.[11] Most hospitals and health systems instead participate in capitation where there is limited health system market power to oppose doing so (i.e., Medicaid managed care markets). Additionally, the increase in quality reporting requirements and emphasis on metrics for participation in other value-based programs has led to a substantial increase in the administrative burden[12] placed on operational leaders.

Finally, the patient-as-consumer movement, in which publicly available ratings and scores are increasingly tied to reimbursement, has compounded these challenges.

In addition to the operational challenges that inhibit expanding and extending student roles, the administrative, financial, and operational actualities of research productivity limits are an additional problem. There is ever-increasing competition for a limited pool of federal grants available to support research efforts as the time to research independence (as measured by receipt of R-series federal grants) increases. This is in the face of growing indirect costs not originally included in NIH grants[13] that now average 52%[14] and increasing pressure to publish scholarly work as a market differentiator.[15] Additionally, faculty time devoted to conducting research due to these operational and financial pressures is decreasing.

Finally, we must mention the educational challenges that stand to impede the growth and sustainability of value-added roles for students. Often, only a fraction of the large number of AMC faculty are integrated, aware, and fully committed to the implementation of curricular changes. Students often report that preceptors and clinical faculty seem disconnected from the intent of their coursework at best and, in the worst of circumstances, outwardly oppose the changes or curricular philosophy.[16] As more institutions work to advance curricular innovations (i.e., use of virtual anatomy tools,[17] problem-based learning, integration of electronic health records, and implementation of telehealth tools), these challenges will be amplified. Additionally, many students increasingly view themselves as consumers rather than learners. All of these characteristics pose substantial challenges to increasing and sustaining the implementation of value-added roles for students.

IMPORTANCE OF STAKEHOLDER PERSPECTIVES

When contemplating expansion and integration of value-added roles for medical students, you will find it helpful to contemplate the differing needs of two key stakeholder groups: faculty and students. Faculty often look for roles that can aid in their efforts to support clinical volume, improve quality, decrease costs, enhance patient satisfaction, and enable the execution of a clinical research agenda (e.g., facilitating patient enrollment in trials). Students, on the other hand, often focus on understanding how they can fulfil the minimum requirements of the required curriculum in order to advance to the next stage of their formal training. The informal or "unspoken" curriculum as noted earlier in the text heavily influences perceptions around the value of participation in activities—required or otherwise—including the value-added roles discussed in this text. Even early in medical school, many students have a clear understanding of their long-term professional directionality, even if they are not settled on specialty choice. This could include a desire to engage in bench or clinical research or to develop health policy, advocacy, management, or entrepreneurship skills. Value-added roles that are sensitive to, and aligned with, the individual needs of students and faculty are more likely to be sustainable.

As discussed elsewhere in several prior chapters, AMCs should contemplate a variety of value-added models, including emphasizing the student as a (1) clinician, (2) researcher, (3) educator, or (4) manager. Many of the examples in this text have emphasized clinical roles, including integrated workflow support to improve clinical volumes, enabling graduated independence over time. Other strategies include carving out specific tasks that often can be assigned early in training, such as serving as an observer, history taker, examiner, or scribe. Additional examples in this text have shared involvement of students in creating value by inclusion in quality support roles or systems redesign.

The authors give limited attention to value-added roles in the research context, but they can be equally valuable. This can include roles in basic science activities, clinical research, and health services and policy research. Roles can range from limited assistance with project management to independent design and execution of a full-fledged project. There are numerous opportunities to provide regulatory support and data analysis, contribute to scholarly writing, or serve as co-contributor to policy development. There are also situations in which value-added roles can be created that link grant development with a democratic "you do the work, you get credit" approach that can involve students in activities including serving as a co-investigator. Many students participate in health systems science projects related to operational analysis of existing workflows; design of new workflows; or projection of operational, customer, and financial impacts. Each of these serves to link front-line clinicians to health system leadership. There have been many examples of students providing value related to policy research and advocacy, including problem scoping; engaging with stakeholders; solution design; direct implementation; or supporting other local, state, and federal actors in implementation.

We need to explicitly mention value-added educational roles for medical students. Due to accreditation requirements, students are often deeply engaged in curricular feedback and redesign. However, a growing number of institutions have enabled students to lead postgraduate surveys of usefulness and/or undertake analysis of how tuition dollars are spent and benefit the customer (i.e., student).

OVERCOMING OBSTACLES: STRATEGIES TO IMPROVE AND GROW VALUE-ADDED ROLES

Given the multitude of challenges facing AMCs, the needs of various stakeholders, and the variety of value-added roles, we now turn to a set of strategies specific to overcoming these obstacles when seeking to improve and grow value-added roles. We contemplate how development of short-term wins, efforts to consolidate gains, evaluation and feedback, and shifting and leveraging culture can all lead to elevating and sustaining change.

Short-Term Wins

We cannot overstate the importance of planning for, achieving, and then celebrating short-term wins. The long-term effort needed to embed and sustain changes in educational approaches over time is massive. These efforts are often threatened by numerous factors that have the potential to derail educational change. By anticipating short-term wins as a part of the overall implementation strategy, it is often possible to emphasize to stakeholders the immediate value of the efforts expended while continuing to drive toward the long-term goal of a sustainable integration, a strategy executed by multiple AMCs.[18]

According to Kotter, there are six key reasons these short-term wins are essential. First, they demonstrate to others that the effort being expended is worth the trouble. Second, they serve to reward those involved by acknowledging their contributions. Third, they assist with adjusting overall strategies as progress is achieved and clarity is obtained about the path forward. Fourth, they limit the ability of others to block further progress. Fifth, they show to stakeholders that implementation is proceeding as planned. Sixth, they enable the project to gain momentum among stakeholders.

While short-term wins are an important tool, they must be planned for and obtained with intentionality, not accident. It is also key to not trade off a short-term win at the expense of a long-term goal or jeopardize the overall approach. Short-term wins lend credibility to the implementation process and give stakeholders confidence to lower lingering opposition.

Consolidating Gains

While short-term wins are important to build momentum, you must be careful not to celebrate too early. Rather, consolidate the gains that have been made and continue to iteratively improve and refine the implementation. If you are too quick to celebrate the short-term wins, you may promote resistance that might not otherwise be evident.

As new approaches to incorporating medical student roles accelerate, you must not let up before the change is fully embedded across the health system or partner organizations. If this occurs, critical momentum is likely to be lost, progress will disappear, and, in the worst case, the project will revert to the original state. New roles for students and novel approaches to integration should be considered unstable advances until they are fully and completely embedded.

It is helpful to keep in mind that change across complex organizations often has multiple dependencies. Placement of a student in a particular setting to perform a specific task, for example, may require adjustment to the workflows of other learners, faculty, staff, and even patients. In most cases, these dependencies create benefits for some but not all groups. In fact, often there are disadvantages or burdens placed on the other groups that are impacted by the change. Understanding these dependencies is important to allow leaders to find ways to incentivize and motivate all stakeholders and groups impacted by the activities.

Evaluation and Feedback

At this point, obtaining feedback and program evaluation to allow iterative improvement is essential. Creating more, not less, change is a hallmark of successful adoption. This enables additional stakeholders to participate in the work, adding momentum as they buy in to the project activities. While iterative change is important, project leaders need to maintain a clear vision of the goals of the activities and not lose focus as changes are made, additional personnel are involved, potential new sites are recruited, or new activities are developed. It is also helpful at this stage to identify the dependencies described earlier, which are not required or critical, with an eye toward elimination. Simplification of the process facilitates long-term adoption, sustainability, and success. Ideally, as further changes are made and incorporated, the project is no longer considered new or novel, but rather the standard approach to how students are learning and contributing.

Shifting and Leveraging Culture

In order to institutionalize new medical student roles, it is important to ensure alignment of the organizational culture with the contributions and activities to facilitate the student roles becoming the norm. New approaches that are inconsistent with organizational values will be difficult to embed and sustain. This may require a shift in culture over time.

Cultural shifts within an organization are possible once new activities occur and individuals have been exposed to the novel approach and experienced the adjustments. Only when these "new" activities become the norm can culture shift. This typically requires a substantial period of time. While slow, these shifts in organizational culture can be transformative because they (1) make use of the collective action of people across the organization, and (2) enable activities to occur without deliberate effort. This reduces the possibility that individuals will obstruct efforts.

Scaling and Sustaining Change

After the successful implementation and long-term adoption of new value-added roles, projects can be scaled to other learners and areas. There are a number of approaches that may be considered when contemplating approaches to scale efforts across other groups. Learning communities may be one helpful tactic. These regular gatherings of project leaders and stakeholders that enable the sharing of experiences in an ongoing conversation can be valuable to sustain momentum and generate greater buy-in outside of the initial project leaders.

Intentional alignment of activities to organizational priorities is also an important tool. For example, if an organization has a shared goal around accelerating patient and community influenza vaccination rates, you could link value-added roles to that objective. Students could engage in quality improvement projects to partner with technology companies to create automated texts and phone calls to unvaccinated patients, work with retail chains to set up community vaccination clinics, or offer vaccination to the families of surgical patients who represent a captive audience while their loved ones are undergoing a procedure.

CONCLUSION

The concepts outlined in this final chapter are designed to help innovators improve and grow value-added roles. Having a deliberate and timely plan for generating short-term wins during implementation, consolidating those gains while beginning evaluation and feedback, and ultimately anchoring these new educational approaches within an organizational culture are likely to be useful approaches. Educators must recognize and emphasize the need to identify and align value-added roles to the student's interests and long-term career objectives. Additionally, tight integration into the clinical workflow is essential to achieve any degree of sustainability. Success requires utilization of both the formal and informal curriculum. Roles that fulfill both are most likely to enable impact.

TAKE-HOME POINTS

1. The current models for financing medical education and supporting academic medical centers are under tremendous financial pressure.
2. Understanding how medical student value-added roles can align with the needs of key stakeholders at institutions is paramount to the long-term sustainability of implementation efforts.
3. Organizations can generate short-term wins during implementation, consolidate those gains while beginning evaluation and feedback, and ultimately anchor these new educational approaches within an organization's culture consistent with the models illustrated by Kotter and Kern.

QUESTIONS FOR FURTHER THOUGHT

1. How can you recognize when a change or new activity has been successfully embedded within the culture of an organization?
2. What additional steps can you take to sustain and scale efforts across other health professions or outside of medicine?

ANNOTATED BIBLIOGRAPHY

Grischkan JA, Friedman AB, Chandra A. Moving the financing of graduate medical education into the 21st century. *JAMA*. 2020;324(11):1035–1036.
This article describes the primary US approach to GME financing that has been in place since the 1980s, describing direct and indirect GME payments. The authors outline how GME training programs can be lucrative for teaching hospitals and why there has been a willingness to expand residency positions without federal funding. The article then describes how GME financing could be reformed to achieve greater benefits for those impacted by the current approach to GME financing.

Gonzalo JD, Lucey C, Wolpaw T, Chang A. Value-added clinical systems learning roles for medical students that transform education and health. *Acad Med*. 2017;92(5):602–607. https://doi.org/10.1097/acm.0000000000001346.
This article provides a very useful overview of Kotter's steps for change management and Kern's steps for curriculum development. The authors provide examples of using these frameworks in the context of incorporating value-added roles for medical students in their respective institutions.

Stimpson JP, Li T, Shiyanbola OO, Jacobson JJ. Financial sustainability of academic health centers: identifying challenges and strategic responses. *Acad Med*. 2014;89(6):853–857.
This article discusses the important role that academic health centers play in training health care personnel and delivering services to the most complex and underresourced patients.

The authors describe the unique financial challenges that academic health centers face and discuss how reforms that have been implemented under the Affordable Care Act create additional downward financial pressure on academic centers. This article provides a helpful review of current challenges and a summary of potential solutions.

REFERENCES

1. Grischkan JA, Friedman AB, Chandra A. Moving the financing of graduate medical education into the 21st century. *JAMA*. 2020;324(11):1035–1036.
2. Stimpson JP, Li T, Shiyanbola OO, Jacobson JJ. Financial sustainability of academic health centers: identifying challenges and strategic responses. *Acad Med*. 2014;89(6):853–857.
3. Kotter JP. *Leading Change*. Boston: Harvard Business School Press; 1996.
4. Thomas PA, Kern DE, Hughes MT, Chen BY. *Curriculum Development for Medical Education: A Six-Step Approach*. 3rd ed. Baltimore, MD: The Johns Hopkins University Press; 2015.
5. Rockey S. Our commitment to supporting the new generation. https://nexus.od.nih.gov/all/2012/02/03/our-commitment-to-supporting-the-next-generation/. Published February 3, 2012. Accessed January 20, 2021.
6. Kesselheim AS, Austed KE. Residents: workers or students in the eyes of the law? *N Engl J Med*. 2011;364:697–699.
7. American Association of Medical Colleges. Advancing the academic health system for the future: a report from the AAMC Advisory Panel on Health Care. 2014. https://www.manatt.com/uploadedFiles/Content/2_Our_People/Enders,_Thomas/AdvancingtheAcademicHealthSystemfortheFuture_AAMC_Mar2014_Paper.PDF. Accessed January 20, 2021.
8. Lopez E, Neuman T, Jacobson G, Levitt L. How much more than medicare do private insurers pay? A review of the literature. *Kaiser Family Foundation*. Published April 15, 2020. Accessed April 24, 2021.
9. Sandson JI. A crisis in medical education: the high cost of student financial assistance. *N Engl J Med*. 1983;308(21):1286–1289.
10. Institute of Medicine of the National Academies. Graduate medical education that meets the nation's health needs. July 2014. https://www.ncbi.nlm.nih.gov/books/NBK248027/pdf/Bookshelf_NBK248027.pdf.
11. James BC, Poulsen GP. The case for capitation. *Harv Bus Rev*. August 2016
12. Wilensky G. The need to simplify measuring quality in health care. *The JAMA Forum*. June 19, 2018
13. National Institutes of Health. NIH history 2020. https://www.nih.gov/about-nih/who-we-are/history. Accessed January 20, 2021.
14. Ledford H. Keeping the lights on. *Nature*. 2014;515:326–329.
15. Budd JM, Stewart KN. Is there such a thing as 'least publishable unit'? An empirical investigation. *Libres*. 2015;25(2):78–85.

16. Wiggleton C, Petrusa E, Loomis K, et al. Medical students' experiences of moral distress: development of a web-based survey. *Acad Med.* 2010;85(1):111–117.

17. Ravindran S. Stanford students use new virtual dissection table to study anatomy. *Mercury News.* June 20, 2011. https://www.mercurynews.com/2011/06/20/stanford-students-use-new-virtual-dissection-table-to-study-anatomy/. Accessed January 20, 2021.

18. Gonzalo JD, Lucey C, Wolpaw T, Chang A. Value-added clinical systems learning roles for medical students that transform education and health. *Acad Med.* 2017;92(5):602–607.

accuracy   One of the standards introduced for strong evaluation in public health. Indicates the degree to which the result of a measurement, calculation, or specification conforms to the correct value or standard.

activities   One of the recommended components of a logic model used for program evaluation. Processes and/or actions used to implement a program.

assessment   Systematic process for gathering and documenting data on the knowledge, skill, attitudes, and beliefs of learners. Used to refine programs and to provide useful feedback about what and how well students are learning.

change agent   A person internal or external to an organization who helps an organization, or part of an organization, transform how it functions.

clinical microsystem   A small, interdependent group of physicians and other health care professionals who work together regularly to provide care for specific groups of patients.

community health center   Community-based and patient-directed organizations that deliver comprehensive, culturally competent, high-quality primary and preventive health care services.

community of practice   Groups of people who share a concern or a passion for something they do and learn how to do it better as they interact regularly.

community oriented primary care (COPC)   A model of primary care that stresses the role of community context in individual health. In COPC, elements of primary health care and community medicine are systematically developed and brought together in a coordinated practice.

equity   The absence of unfair and avoidable or remediable differences in health outcomes among population groups that are defined socially, economically, demographically, or geographically.

evaluation   The systematic use of a variety of methods to collect, analyze, and use information to determine whether a program is fulfilling its mission(s) and achieving its goal(s).

evaluation plan   A living document that describes how a program will be monitored and evaluated, as well as how evaluation results will be used for program improvement and decision-making.

feasibility   One of the standards introduced for strong evaluation in public health. Refers to the degree that something can be easily or conveniently done or how realistic, prudent, diplomatic, and frugal an approach is.

federally qualified community health center   A specific type of community health center, in which community-based health care providers receive funds from the Health Resources and Services Administration Health Center Program to provide primary care services in underserved areas.

gap analysis   Compares actual performance with what was expected or desired. In health care, it clarifies the discrepancy between current reality and the desired or optimal health care situation and identifies an opportunity that may be addressed.

health systems science   A foundational platform and framework for the study and understanding of how care is delivered, how health professionals work together to deliver that care, and how the health system can improve patient care and health care delivery.

impacts   One of the recommended components of a logic model used for program evaluation. Refers to measurable changes that occur as a result of program implementation.

inputs   One of the recommended components of a logic model used for program evaluation. Refers to resources used to implement a program; may include financial, physical, and/or human resources.

Institute for Healthcare Improvement (IHI) Model for Improvement   A framework to guide improvement work, focusing on changes on a small scale using Plan-Do-Study-Act (PDSA) cycles.

Lean A3 template   A standardized health care continuous improvement tool originally developed by and for the Toyota Motor Corporation to document and track improvements in manufacturing processes.

Lean methodology   A systematic method of eliminating waste focused on activity that adds value. Originally developed by Toyota.

logic model   An action-oriented tool used for program evaluation and strategic reporting activities. The Centers for Disease Control and Prevention defines a logic model as "a graphic depiction (road map) that presents the shared relationships among the resources, activities, outputs, outcomes, and impact for your program."

macrosystems   The container that holds meso- and microsystems together in the health system, such as a hospital or large health center.

mesosystem   Interlinked system of microsystems in which a person participates. In health care, mesosystems link microsystems, allowing patients and care personnel to move among disparate units and to support patients along their continuum of care.

microsystem   A small group of professionals who work together on a regular basis, or as needed, to provide care to discrete populations of patients.

mixed methods   An evaluation method that combines elements from both quantitative and qualitative approaches, which can be complementary to one another.

National Academy of Medicine six aims of quality health care   An analytic framework for quality assessment that can guide and measure development initiatives in the public and private sectors. States that health care should be safe, effective, patient centered, timely, efficient, and equitable.

outcomes   One of the recommended components of a logic model used for program evaluation. Refers to the results used to determine whether a program met its anticipated goals; can be short term, intermediate, or long term.

outputs   One of the recommended components of a logic model used for program evaluation. Refers to the products of program activities.

patient navigator   A distinct role on a health care team. The key principles of patient navigation include focusing care on patients and their needs, integrating access to resources to meet the needs of patients interacting with a fragmented system, seeking to eliminate or prevent barriers, facilitating care across sites and locations, and coordinating care.

Plan-Do-Study-Act (PDSA)   Part of the Institute for Healthcare Improvement's Model for Improvement. Steps in the PDSA cycle:

Step 1: Plan—Plan the test or observation, including a plan for collecting data.

Step 2: Do—Try out the test.

Step 3: Study—Set aside time to analyze the data and study the results.

Step 4: Act—Refine the change based on what was learned from the test.

propriety   One of the standards introduced for strong evaluation in public health. The quality or state of being proper or suitable, it incorporates legal and ethical behavior at all times, with regard for the welfare of those involved and those affected.

qualitative methods   Used to acquire information that answers questions regarding process, value, and accountability, some of which may be difficult to quantify. Qualitative measures answer questions that are open ended rather than discrete. The data can be captured from observations, interviews, case studies, or focus groups.

quality improvement   The combined and unceasing efforts of health care professionals, patients, their families, researchers, payers, planners, and educators to make changes that will lead to better patient outcomes, better system performance, and better professional development.

quantitative methods   Provide numeric, countable data that can be used to measure outputs and quantify impact. Data can be collected from surveys, assessments, questionnaires, exams, rubrics, and other data collection instruments.

service learning   Education involving programs that engage students and staff in actual service delivery. Services provided range from primary care and preventive services to broader community development and mobilization.

social determinants of health   The conditions in which people are born, grow, live, work, and age, which affect a wide range of health, functioning, and quality-of-life outcomes and risks. Five key areas include economic stability, education, social and community context, health and health care, and neighborhood and built environment.

systems thinking   Recognizing and understanding the complex interdependencies and relationships within a functional system such as health care. Allows the formation of linkages among disparate areas of activity in health care to improve outcomes, patient experience, and value in health care.

utility   One of the standards introduced for strong evaluation in public health. Refers to the way in which information collected will serve the needs of the intended users.

value-added roles   Designed to provide students with opportunities to engage in health systems science and clinical skills while adding value to the health care system by legitimately contributing to patient care. Alternate definition: Experiential roles for students in practice environments that have the potential to positively impact individual patient and population health outcomes, costs of care, or other processes within the health system while also enhancing student knowledge, attitudes, and skills in the clinical or health systems sciences.

Page numbers followed by "*f*" indicate figures, "*t*" indicate tables, and "*b*" indicate boxes.